WEAR MORE

cashmere

WEAR MORE
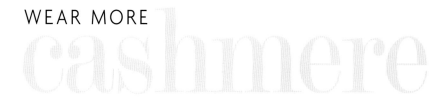

151 LUXURIOUS WAYS TO
PAMPER YOUR INNER PRINCESS

by Jennifer "Gin" Sander

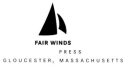

FAIR WINDS
PRESS
GLOUCESTER, MASSACHUSETTS

Text © 2003, 2005 by Jennifer "Gin" Sander

First published in the USA in 2003 by
Fair Winds Press
33 Commercial Street
Gloucester, MA 01930

First edition published 2003.
Paperback edition published 2005.

08 07 06 05   1 2 3 4 5

ISBN 1-59233-142-4

Library of Congress Cataloging-in-Publication Data available

Cover and interior design by Laura McFadden
Cover and interior illustrations by Steven Salerno

Printed and bound in China

The chocolate pudding recipe on page 30 reprinted with
permission from Elaine Corn. Copyright © 1994, Elaine Corn.
Lobster Bisque recipe on page 72 excerpted from *Silver Palate Good
Times Cookbook*. Copyright © 1984, 1985 by Julee Rosso and Sheila
Lukins. Used by permission of Workman Publishing Co., Inc.,
New York. All rights reserved.

*Dedicated to the memory—not to mention
the style—of Diana Vreeland.*

by Gin Sander

YEARS AGO I STUCK A MINI POST-IT ON THE side of my computer that read "Wear more cashmere." It was a little reminder to myself, a fairly new wife and a brand-new mother, that I needed to spend a little time on myself, more often than I'd been doing. Yes, I deserved to wear more cashmere, deserved to feel the lovely warmth and softness of that tightly woven fabric sliding on my skin. "Wear more cashmere" was my way of telling myself this—that I deserved a few minutes to myself in which I could relax in a hot bath without a knock on the door. Why did I need to remind myself of this, when it seems so obvious? It does indeed seem obvious, but the fact is that almost every woman I know spreads herself dangerously thin without allowing herself these little personal luxuries every so often. Let's review the list: There is my husband, my children, my work, my kitchen, my house, my garden—everything needs my attention but *me*. I'm last on my list, and I'm guessing you show up last on *your* list, too.

So I decided to take matters into my own hands and make sure that there were moments in my life when I felt special. The moments might not happen every hour, but maybe only every few days, and certainly every few weeks.

Understand this: No one will just hand you the luxurious and self-indulgent life you dream of. It won't happen unless you make it happen on your own. So why sit there waiting? Pick up your princess self, get out there, and get started. Don't wait passively to be "asked" to do anything, whether you are waiting to be asked to some fancy-dress occasion or to an elegant cocktail party. Why wait? Invite *yourself*. Make it happen. Tell yourself it is perfectly okay to reward yourself with any one of the 150-plus treats that await you in this book. Sometimes it may be as simple and easy as ordering champagne instead of chardonnay before dinner. You can do that, can't you?

Now then, where does all of this "princess" stuff come from? A princess? Not a real princess, mind you. I once had the good fortune to be mistaken for a real princess (true story, ladies) for five days. Trust me on this, five days was enough. Maybe a little too long, I thought, by the fifth day. As Princess Diana learned, too, a life of endless shopping is dreadfully dull.

I'm not encouraging you to be a helpless, simpering, silly thing, unable to turn on a light switch. That is not what I mean by your inner princess.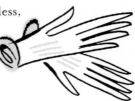

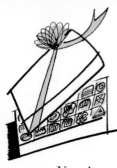 Yes, your inner princess. That deep longing each and every one of us has, to feel that we are truly different from those around us, worthy of being pampered and cared for and fussed over.

You do not want others to treat you like a princess, however. If they did, you would feel utterly alone, trust no one, and never really know who your friends were. Be realistic—the most any of us can aspire to are fleeting moments of luxury, indulgence, and ease. Once or twice my house has been featured in lifestyle magazines, but does that mean it always looks picture-perfect? Does that mean that I don't have to pick up Dr. Pepper cans and small boys' underpants from every room, all throughout the day? For the last magazine shoot, three people worked non-stop for a week to make the house perfect for the photos. The minute the photographers pulled out of the driveway, it was back to life as usual, soda cans, underpants, and all. I also hung around a friend's house once, when *Martha Stewart Living* was photographing her life...holding back my snickers at how temporarily perfect it all appeared. So if your house, or your life, doesn't look picture-perfect, don't despair. We're doing fine if we can capture a moment of beauty and fleeting perfection. Create one tiny corner of your life where you can sit and believe that all is right with the world.

There will be days like this, your own mother might have told you, as she sipped a cup of tea and gazed out the window at the gloomy weather. Days when you will need a little something extra to feel loved, days when you'll dare to indulge your own deep desire to look like a star, and nights when you will long for a touch of

specialness. Days when you wish you could wear more cashmere...Coco Chanel knew how to feel special on days like that.
Dead broke and shivering on the French coast, she slipped into her
boyfriend's oversized sweater and started a fashion trend. Why not
learn how to adopt a small, stylish gesture that will make you feel
like a million dollars on the inside? Soon you, too, will be turn-
ing heads and starting trends as you move regally through life.

Four women of enormous style—who certainly wore cashmere
more often than the ordinary women of their day—are Diana
Vreeland, Coco Chanel, Wallis Windsor, and Jacqueline
Kennedy Onassis. You will see them quoted often
in the following pages. These four are my
"luxury role models," women whose lives have
been filled with style and glamour. Okay, so
they also had a lot of cash. But not everything they did takes tons of money to
do—does it cost any money to sit up
straighter and move with grace? To hold
yourself as though you were indeed a princess? To create a
signature look—a slash of red lipstick in Ms. Vreeland's case, or
Ms. Chanel's borrowed menswear? No. These, and many other
ways of indulging yourself in grand style, cost little or nothing.

Long before she became the famous and flamboyant editor of
Vogue magazine, Diana Vreeland began to write a column for
Harper's Bazaar called "Why Don't You..." in which she made
whimsical suggestions to readers about things they should try.
"Why don't you...wash your blonde children's hair in dead
champagne, as they do in France?" was one of her more

memorable suggestions. Or this one: "Why don't you...turn your old ermine coat into a bathrobe?" Why not, indeed. I heard Ms. Vreeland's distinctive voice in my ear as I wrote much of *Wear More Cashmere.* I am encouraging you to try whimsical and creative things that will make you feel like the special woman that you are. I'm hoping they are a teeny bit more practical than the ermine bathrobe idea (but really, *wouldn't* that feel great?).

In the beautifully designed pages of *Wear More Cashmere: 151 Luxurious Ways to Pamper Your Inner Princess,* you'll find page after page of ideas to make your humdrum everyday life a tiny bit more indulgent. Not more expensive, mind you. This book isn't about spending pots of money on useless things. It is about spending time (okay, and maybe a little bit of money) creating a different world for yourself. A private world, unlike the hard-edged and fast-paced one we move through most of the day.

Wear More Cashmere will teach you simple ways to:

- **Feel special.** Slip into bed and feel your skin surrounded by the smoothness of high-count cotton sheets.
- **Look special.** Step into a pair of mules and adopt that forties glamour-girl air.
- **Be special.** Grow pale-pink orchids in your bathroom, an uncommonly luxurious hobby to acquire, or invent a cocktail of your own—named after you, of course.

I'm hoping this book will be a delightful luxury object in itself, designed to make any woman holding it feel that she *is* royalty, ready to be coddled and pampered and have her every whim catered to by a cast of thousands. So sit back on your throne (see idea # 25), and start reading.

Enjoy!
JENNIFER "GIN" SANDER
GRANITE BAY, CALIFORNIA

forties glamour and some mules

WOULD YOU LIKE TO TRANSFORM YOURSELF quickly into a woman of glamour and mystery? Slip into a pair of mules—those old-fashioned, high-heeled backless slippers. Instant forties movie-star glamour and sex appeal, guaranteed. You will suddenly view the world as a place in which you are petted and pampered. What is it about a pair of high-heeled mules that can give you that Joan Crawford kind of feeling? Is it that slappy sound as you sashay down the hallway? Is it the sexy way you can cross your legs and then dangle one shoe in a sassy manner? I'm not sure what it is about mules, but it works every time. Add a pair of mules to your everyday uniform of jeans and a t-shirt, and you will feel like a completely different woman, the sort of woman who lives in a penthouse apartment and drives a Jag. ⚭

counting sheep

ONE OF LIFE'S TRUE LUXURIES IS A GOOD NIGHT'S SLEEP, A LUXURY that seems to slip through our fingers more often than not in today's world. So why not reward yourself with a good night's sleep as often as possible? Many things in this book will combine to make your bedroom a place of repose and relaxation. I'll start off with just one such little luxury. Adding one simple thing to your bedtime routine—wearing wool socks to bed—can help tremendously. I'll spare you the scientific details (while pretending to understand them myself), but it has something to do with regulating the body's temperature. So find yourself the most luxurious, most expensive socks you can (yes, there are even cashmere socks), and you will enjoy true indulgence at night for less than $30. Aren't you smart and cozy? Sounds goofy, I know, but take it from someone who does not fall asleep easily...it works! ∂

silky smooth

AH, THE FEELING OF SLEEK AND GLOSSY SKIN, THE GENTLE WHIFF of your favorite perfume, but those bath oils can be so beastly dear in price. Instead of spending your money on expensive bath oils, why not just make your own? For many years I would pour plain old baby oil into my hot bath and then add a few drops of my current favorite perfume. It wasn't until I read the auto-biography of famed *Vogue* editor Diana Vreeland that I learned this was foolish. She describes one wealthy young woman who would dump the entire contents of an expensive bottle of perfume into her tub: "Of course you don't get anything out of a tub with perfume in it—it has no oil in it, only alcohol. This was just a gesture of glory, she was madly extrav-agant." Perfume merely dissipates in hot water, but it "binds" to oil. So instead of wasting your perfume in a madly extravagant gesture, here is what you should do. First pour some baby oil into a small cup, *then* add a few drops of your perfume into the oil. Swish it around, *then* pour it into the tub! The oil won't evaporate away, and it holds the perfume scent for you. Float a few fresh-cut flowers around for an extra touch of glamour. Just don't forget to clean up the oil afterward with a bit of cleansing powder on the floor of your tub, lest you slip and fall on your princess behind the next time you stand up in your shower. ⚶

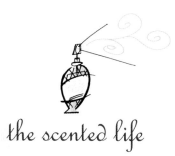

the scented life

I LOVE THE SMELL OF PERFUME, BUT THE ACTUAL COST OF PERFUME can sometimes make me gag. Thankfully, the perfume industry has provided us with a way to bring their lovely scents into our lives for less. Every magazine comes stuffed with a perfume insert, or two or three. *Tell* me you don't toss old magazines into the trash without ripping those pages out! No, dear, rip them out immediately, open, and fill your life with expensive scents. Yes, you could rub them on your wrist for a thrill that will last an hour or so, but I like to put them to work for longer periods of time. I regularly put sample scent strips into my underwear drawer and sometimes tuck them under my pillow (only on your side of the bed, though, as men aren't always that fond of sleeping in a heavily perfumed room). Other less romantic uses are to uncover a strip and stash it in your car, somewhere it won't be seen but can still be smelled. I even tuck one discreetly in the trash can of the guest bathroom before my friends arrive. The scent won't last forever, but for a few days, anyway, your underwear, your car, or the inside of your handbag can smell like $150 an ounce—until next month's issue of a fashion magazine arrives in the mail and supplies you with fresh new scents. ❧

the high life

AH, ONE OF LIFE'S MOST PERFECT MOMENTS...NO, NOT AS YOU step down the aisle as a dreamy bride, not when you discover you are holding the winning lottery numbers. I mean the moment that you slip between the coolness of high-count cotton sheets. High thread count, that is. Try it just once, and you will never go back. By high thread count I mean 250 plus...300 and above is even better. Yes, they are pricey. And I want you to be able to sleep at night guilt-free, so please don't rush out and spend hundreds and hundreds on a set of Egyptian cotton. I hunt on the bargain tables of retail companies like Tuesday Morning, Ross, or Marshalls to find deals on these expensive sheets. Outlet stores like Ralph Lauren also have marked-down expensive sheets in a back corner. The secret to a long and happy marriage is in the sheets. Not satin, not silk, but high-count cotton. ᴧ

indulge your dreams

EVERY NIGHT WHEN YOU CLOSE YOUR EYES AND DREAM, AN INCREDIBLE thing happens: You become a writer, director, producer, wardrobe manager, scenery director, and location scout, effortlessly producing mini-movies all night long. Wouldn't it be wonderful if you could tap into one-tenth of that creativity during your waking hours? But alas, even the most vivid dreams fade after a few hours—unless, of course, you write them down.

Create a beautiful dream journal. Buy the fanciest, most gold-encrusted portfolio there is, and fill its pages with your own dream productions. Every morning upon waking, instead of rushing off to jump under a shocking shower, allow yourself to stay in your warm little nest and run back over what your mind produced the night before. Don't struggle with trying to understand them; this is not analysis. It is merely a record of what your own luxurious imagination is capable of producing when you aren't watching. And the more you accumulate waking evidence of what your mind can produce, the more confident you'll be when you need to tap into your creativity during work hours. ⟨⟩

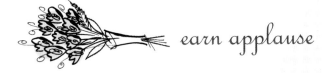 earn applause

SADLY, THERE ISN'T MUCH BOWING AND CURTSEYING GOING ON nowadays, making us feel special and acknowledged as we enter a room. Sigh. But there is still a little something that can make you feel like a princess upon entering a room—applause. Trust me, the sight and sound of a roomful of people clapping for *you* is amazing. So you need to immediately get involved in some kind of pursuit that is likely to lead to applause. Do something, *anything*, that will regularly allow you to hear yourself applauded. Amateur acting, singing, performing, anything for which a group of people will look at you with beaming faces and start to clap on your behalf. Regular applause is not as hard to arrange as you might imagine. A few years ago, I joined the speaking club Toastmasters International in order to work on my public speaking skills. Sounds scary, but try it! Every time you are introduced and stand at a meeting, the clapping starts. Maybe there is a chapter near you? Visit www.toastmasters.org to find out. ꙮ

ready for your close-up?

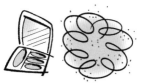

MODELS IN MAGAZINES LOOK BEAUTIFUL AND PERFECT SIMPLY because, before the photo was shot, someone spent hours doing their hair, their makeup, their clothes. They didn't show up for the shoot looking that way. So why not treat yourself to that same kind of experience, where you can be fussed over like a super-model, if only for a few hours? Spend the time, spend the money, on a glamour shot. Okay, so the models are being paid to go through that, whereas you will have to pay to have the same experience. But trust me, it is worth it—not only for the feeling of being fussed over, but also for the end result: a professional photo that captures a moment in time when you did look per-fect (because you were wearing ten times as much makeup as you ordinarily would, your hair was lacquered within an inch of its life, and you were holding a bizarre and awkward pose). And once you have treated yourself to a day of professional makeup and photography, you will never again feel intimidated or inadequate when you look at a model in a magazine, because you'll know exactly how long it took to create that perfect look. Keep the photo on your desk to remind yourself (and your friends, family, and coworkers) just what a glamorous girl you really are. ⚭

candlelight oasis

AN INDULGENT WAY TO SPEND AN EVENING ALONE IS TO TURN YOUR
own bedroom into a candlelight palace. No, not for a lover, just
for yourself. Place scented candles all around the room, group
them in strategic corners (away from the draperies, please), and
create a glamorous and cozy lair in which to sit back and read in
bed. Reading in bed undisturbed is truly one of a woman's greatest luxuries. You might choose books about women who lived
with great style and flair—perhaps Diana Vreeland's auto-
biography, *D.V.*, a particular favorite of mine. Or *The Power of Style*,
by Annette Tapert and Diana Edkins. Who wouldn't enjoy whiling
away an hour or two reading about the lives of wealthy style
queens from days past, such as Babe Paley, Slim Keith, and
Jacqueline Kennedy Onassis? We rarely get to
enter the world of privilege for just the cost of
a book and a lazy, candlelit evening alone. ⋀

hitting a high note

LOVELY AS IT IS TO RECEIVE A HANDWRITTEN NOTE IN THE MAIL from a friend, it is just as enjoyable to sit down and write one yourself. Who needs a reason? Formal thank-you notes are always welcome, but just as fun to indulge in are little personal notes to tell friends about a movie they might enjoy, or to enclose a clipped article that might be of interest. As we all shift to e-mail, faxes, and computerized correspondence, think of how treasured and rare handwritten letters have become. Indulge in a box of high-quality personalized stationery or note cards, such as beautiful paper with pretty flowered lining on the inside of the envelope, and don't forget your impressive gold-stamped monogram! It is such a delicious feeling to hold one of those stiff cards in your hand, affix a stamp carefully in the upper-right corner, and walk it to the mailbox. Makes you feel like a heroine in a Jane Austen novel, doesn't it? As with so many aspects of life (love, money, kindness), what you put out there comes back to you manyfold. The more lovely letters you drop in the mail, the greater the chances that your mailbox will soon be overflowing in turn. ⟨♠⟩

reading beyond your means

NO DOUBT YOU KNOW THE TROUBLESOME PHRASE "LIVING BEYOND your means," and the disaster and peril that await those who do. I am sternly in favor of living within your means, but I am equally in favor of what I call "reading beyond your means." It only costs a few dollars to buy a copy of *Architectural Digest*, *Town & Country*, or *Gourmet*. It costs millions to try to imitate the lifestyles shown within. Go ahead and indulge yourself with a few hours of peeking in on the lifestyles of the very, very rich. Don't use this as an excuse to get all worked up about your lot in life; don't march out and charge something you saw advertised and saddle yourself with years of debt. Do pay attention to the smaller things—the colors the rooms are painted in a palace, for instance. Most of us can't really afford the jewelry, the clothes, or the restaurants, but you can find so much about living gracefully, about incorporating beauty and style into your own abode. Over the years I've turned many a fancy photo spread in a magazine into homemade art by cutting up the swanky ads and using them in decoupage projects. I've made picture frames decorated all over with paper cut outs of diamonds and pearls, glued travel photos to the sides of leather suitcases, and covered stained and worn tabletops with my own designs pressed under plexiglass. It is an inexpensive way to bring a bit of *Architectural Digest* gloss into your life. ❦

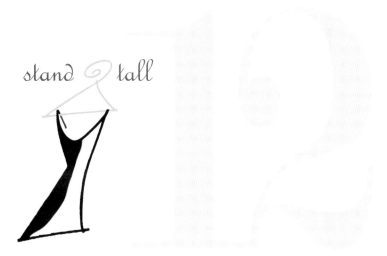

stand tall

HAVE YOU EVER SEEN A WOMAN WHO REALLY STANDS OUT IN a crowded room simply because she looks as if she is somebody? Chances are she was standing up nice and straight. If you want to move through life like a princess, you'd better learn to stand like one. Take a ballet class, regardless of your age. What better way to learn to stand tall and erect than at the barre? And remember that trick with the book on your head? It really works. Stand up and balance a book on your head and walk across the room, carefully placing one foot in front of the other. Then practice sitting and getting in and out of cars. So few of us, myself included, feel comfortable and graceful when clambering out of the back of a car. An observer once said of Evangeline Bruce, the wife of a famed diplomat, that she was "poetry in motion, even in the smallest gestures. She would sink down into one of her Louis XV fauteuils in one graceful movement, her back straight against the chair, one leg folded over the other at the knees...." Are you poetry in motion? If not, then close the curtains in your room, draw yourself up to your fullest height, suck in your tummy, and practice away. ⚭

chocolate cashmere

CHOCOLATE CASHMERE? SOUNDS A BIT HARD TO swallow, literally. But what I mean is this—that you should know how to make a thing or two that melts on your tongue in the same way that cashmere melts on your body. And I believe that home-made chocolate pudding is chocolate cashmere indeed. How indulged can you feel eating lowfat yogurt all the time? Every so often you need to cut loose and let your tongue linger over the honest-to-goodness taste and feel of real fat. I eat real chocolate pudding straight out of the pot, and I think you'll soon do it, too. This recipe is from a wonderful cookbook called *Gooey Desserts*, by Elaine Corn.

Here are the ingredients, and don't you dare go looking for fat-free substitutes for any of them:

Chocolate Pudding from Gooey Desserts

3 egg yolks
1 whole egg
1 cup sugar
3 tablespoons flour
3 tablespoons cocoa
2 cups whole milk
2 tablespoons pure vanilla extract
3 tablespoons butter

I recommend using the most expensive cocoa you can get your hands on, as a lovely little indulgence. Your first step is to beat the yolks and the whole egg together and set that bowl aside. Whisk the sugar, flour, cocoa, and milk in a medium saucepan until the mixture is smooth and lump-free. Turn on the heat to medium and cook the chocolate mixture, stirring all the while, until just under a boil. Remove it from the stove, and whisk in the egg mixture very quickly and very well. Put the pan back on the stove and, while stirring constantly, continue to cook for another minute or so until it is lovely and thick. Remove it from the heat and then whisk in the vanilla and the butter. Sinfully rich and luxurious. ❧

light your own fire

PICTURE THIS RESTFUL SCENE: YOU CURLED UP WITH A GOOD BOOK, on a deep soft rug, in front of a roaring fire. Mmmm...but wait. Where is the guy who built the fire? Let's face it, princesses can take care of themselves. They don't always have a retinue hanging around to do their bidding. Learn to build a fire yourself, my dear, and you will never again be cold. I confess, it has taken me years to work up the nerve to build a fire without a man around to supervise. And yes, I follow my husband Peter's instructions carefully: Gather up some newspaper, kindling, and logs. Place two logs across the fireplace with about six inches in between. Twist three or four pieces of newspaper lengthwise (Peter thinks the *New York Observer* burns the best), and tuck them between the big logs. Set four or five pieces of kindling crosswise over the logs, and add a log or two of kindling. Light the paper at both ends and snuggle in your jammies in front of a fire you built yourself. If this all sounds confusing, use this as an opportunity to invite someone over to show you how *he* builds a fire. ⟨♫⟩

tailor made

HAND-TAILORED CLOTHES SOUND SO LUXURIOUS, DON'T THEY? And a custom-designed dress? Who could afford that? Well, I think you can, dearie. No matter how small the item—even if you just have a small pair of shorts made—you should once in your life have a piece of clothing that is made for only you. Just for you, no one else. Never will you see it on a rival. Imagine the pleasure you'll get from saying, "Oh this? I had it made." Years ago I had a pair of pants made in Bangkok for the underwhelming sum of $30, much less than the cost of the pair I was having the tailor copy. But I have gotten thousands of dollars' worth of thrills from the way it makes me feel to know that I am moving through life in a pair of pants in the color I wanted in the style I wanted, and cut just for my body. Not off the store rack like every other girl's, these pants are mine alone. Yes, buying custom-made clothing sounds so swanky, but look at a few of the prices—they aren't that much more than a top-of-the-line department store purchase. For those who don't live near an area with tailors in town, check out Shirtcreations by Arthur Gluck, a New York custom shirtmaker (www.shirtcreations.com). A high-quality cotton women's shirt made from custom measurements will run around $150, a silk blouse in the $200 range. ⋏

pearls of wisdom

JEWELS, WHAT COULD BE BETTER? LOVELY DIAMONDS, EMERALDS, and rubies. But with such huge price tags, it is easy to feel left out of the jewel race. Don't despair, there is one classic piece of jewelry that you can indeed afford, and probably from the finest maker. I'm talking about pearls, those legendary gifts from the sea. Celebrated for their purity, reputed to hold healing powers, pearls are for every woman. A simple pair of pearl studs is the ultimate in luxurious accessories. So simple, yet so elegant, it is the only piece of jewelry you ever need to own. And why not go straight to the top—to Tiffany & Company? At Tiffany, the top-of-the-line pearl studs, designed by Jean Schlumberger, are an eye-popping thousand dollars, but a simple pair of pearl studs is $275. Think about it, if you just skip one weekend vacation you can feel so very refined, like Grace Kelly out on an afternoon jaunt. ✍

tie one on

I DIVIDE WOMEN INTO TWO CATEGORIES—THOSE WHO KNOW HOW to wear scarves, and those who don't. For much of my adult life, I was one of the women who didn't. And then I decided to transform myself into one of the women who did. Try it, and see how it makes you feel. Add a silk scarf to your regular blazer, or tie one casually onto the side of your purse or your briefcase. (That style was started by Babe Paley, the wife of CBS owner Bill Paley. She took hers off and tied it to her handbag, photographers snapped the scene, and within weeks everyone was doing it.)

Would you like to feel like Grace Kelly in the movie *To Catch a Thief*? Tie a scarf on your head, don your biggest sunglasses, drive with the top down, and let passersby wonder, "Who *was* that woman?" My own mother once startled us all in the mid-seventies by climbing up on the back of a rented convertible in Hawaii, where she at once began to wave like a beauty queen. And sure enough, folks smiled and waved back at her. Act like a star, and you will be treated like one. The best silk scarves are, of course, from Hermés. And they cost upwards of $300. But type the word "Hermés" into the search function of eBay, and you'll be delighted at what comes up. ⚭

feet first

A TRUE PRINCESS WOULD HAVE MANY ATTENDANTS TO, UM, ATTEND to her. Not the lifestyle we usually get to live now, is it? But there is a way you can spend at least one hour feeling very well attended to indeed. An hour in which you will feel petted and stroked, and you will even get to sit on a throne. Have you guessed? Yes, it is a pedicure. I'll take a pedicure over a manicure any day. It is far more indulgent, and the results ast longer— weeks and weeks for a pedicure, versus the mere days that you get out of even the best manicure before it starts to chip a bit. There you are, relaxed in your salon throne, the manicurist working away to transform your tired feet into elegant and well-cared-for objects. Close your eyes and enjoy the foot massage. I always offer to pay a tiny bit more for a longer foot massage. Such luxury for a scant $20. Not only do you end up with pretty feet, but you are so much more relaxed from the pampering and the effects of the foot massage on those sensitive parts of your feet. Truly a moment to savor. ♠

start drinking stars

WHEN EVERYONE AROUND YOU IS ORDERING SILLY pink cocktails, why not order champagne? After all, it is an aperitif, which makes it perfectly acceptable (and perfectly indulgent) to drink before your meal. For a Gatsbyesque touch, startle your waiter (they do need startling once in a while) and impress your friends with your insouciance by ordering up a glass of French champagne. The delightful thing about champagne is that it isn't nearly as bewildering to order as wine. Just ask for a glass of something recognizable like Bollinger (the brand James Bond drinks), Veuve Clicquot, or Cristal from Louis Roederer. That nice Benedictine monk, Dom Perignon, who invented champagne, did princesses a favor by developing a drink that looks like liquid diamonds. Why wait for a celebratory occasion?

drive, she said

OUR CARS ARE SO MUCH OF OUR PERSONALITIES AND SELF-IMAGE. Why not stake out a new image of indulgence for yourself by tooling around town in an old classic car? That does sound expensive, doesn't it? But it really isn't. A stylish Jag or Mercedes from the seventies can be had for less than $10,000. Imagine the style and dash you will exude with that look! If you don't want to take a chance on an old car, you can always have a day of style and dash by renting a luxurious new car. Hertz rents flashy new Jaguars for around $125 a day, and Avis will send you off the rental lot in a new Cadillac de Ville for less than $100. I rented a Jaguar for three days in the midst of a humdrum business trip to Seattle, and I did feel like a princess. Seems extravagant, but the total cost is nothing compared to what it would cost if you went in over your head and leased one of these pretty puppies. A word to the wise, though—please don't waste your money renting some tacky limo (but never turn it down if someone sends one for you). Nice as it is to have someone else drive you around, it never really feels like an authentic experience, and no one who sees you pass by believes for one minute that that is your car. Kind of takes the fun out of it, doesn't it? .&

don your robes

THE DOORBELL RINGS, AND YOU OPEN THE DOOR SLOWLY TO welcome your caller. Imagine their surprise when they discover you aren't wearing ordinary clothes, but rather a silky caftan robe! "Oh," you'll explain, "I always change when I get home for the day." Sound too wild for you? But think about it. Why not have a sartorial signal to tell yourself that one part of your day—the work part—is now over, and the next part—the relaxing part—can begin? I don't mean a scruffy bathrobe, mind you, but a truly luxurious caftan or robe you wouldn't mind being seen in by friends and family. In the 1920s, famed California architect Bernard Maybeck startled polite society by insisting on wearing only one thing in the sanctuary of his own home: a red velvet robe he designed himself. He designed one for his wife, too, the nice man. The most beautiful robe I ever wore was a heavy brown, gold, and orange woven silk man's robe of Middle Eastern design, which I would slip into when visiting the home of an Arab prince. I always begged my friend to please let me take it home, but no. "I can't give it to you, it isn't mine," he finally admitted. "It belongs to the Sultan of Oman." Oh. A wonderful source of exotic robes that reek of mystery and sophistication is the J. Peterman catalog (www.jpeterman.com). Legendary socialite Daisy Fellowes greeted her guests in leopard-print silk pajamas. What will *you* wear when you come to the door? ∿

a little classy, a little trashy...

WE SPEND SO MUCH OF OUR DAYS AND NIGHTS WORRYING ABOUT making mistakes and social faux pas. Why not just go ahead and do it intentionally? Relax and have a little fun by adding a touch of trampiness to your ordinary outfit. Ignore rules of jewelry;

wear ropes of pearls with your jeans, like Coco Chanel, who wore pearls while riding. Her big ropes of pearls were fake, of course, which adds a bit to their trashiness. But what fun that would be! Here is the secret: As long as you *know* the social rule (no diamonds before 5 P.M., say, or no white after Labor Day), you can choose to openly flout it and impress people with your daring. If you *don't* know the rule and break it, you look like a rube. If you *do* know the rule and break it, you are the ultimate sophisticate. Diana Vreeland said, "a little bad taste is like a nice splash of paprika...*no* taste is what I'm against." So go ahead and add a leopard-print scarf to your sedate blue business suit. Go ahead and wear silky underthings while helping out in your child's kindergarten class—it can be your little secret! ⚭

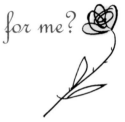

for me?

WHAT WOMAN'S HEART DOESN'T LEAP AT THE SIGHT OF A FLOWER-delivery boy? Most men, however, seem to lack the flower-sending gene. So why wait? Buy fresh flowers for yourself—big bunches of lush and fragrant blooms to brighten your day whenever you need it most. It does sounds lavish and expensive, but it doesn't have to be. Just buy the occasional bunch to put on your desk for a wonderful boost, or grow a cutting garden at home. I buy bunches of white lilianthus, and they last for weeks, which works out to about $1.75 a day. Don't you deserve that? Of course you do. I know I'm worth $1.75 a day, and so are you! The whole point is to go ahead and decide to celebrate yourself, without waiting for anyone else to do it for you. Buy your favorite flower as often as you feel like it, and do not ever feel guilty. ⚘

sweep into a room

QUEEN ELIZABETH MIGHT LOOK A TAD SILLY IN THAT RED VELVET robe with the ermine trim, but those royals do know one thing— put a cape on your shoulders, and your personality is transformed. The glamorous feeling of sweeping down the street in a flowing cloak, or tossing the stray end of a sumptuous shawl over one shoulder, is divine, simply divine.

Get yourself a full-length cape, or a generous-sized shawl, to throw dramatically over your shoulder during critical moments. Yes, for this one you will have to spend a little money, but trust me, it will be well worth it. A catalog company called Art & Artifact sells a burgundy velvet cape for $159, so check out their Web site at www.artandartifact.com. Better yet, have one made. Perhaps this could be the one custom-made article you invest in—a great sweeping cape made of the richest velvet you can find, in the color that most flatters your blue-blooded coloring. ❧

you may enter...

ALL RIGHT, NOW I'M *REALLY* GOING TO ENCOURAGE YOUR delusions of personal grandeur—why not create a throne room or reception area for yourself? No, it doesn't really need to be carved from mahogany and encrusted with gold; a nice comfortable chair that is *yours* and yours alone will do. Paint the walls around it a soft and flattering color. (I once planned to paint my bedroom a deep yellow that I thought would look cheerful. "Oh dear..." my mother said, "yellow does not flatter a woman's complexion first thing in the morning." She was right. I painted it rose instead.) And angle the lights in the room to make sure you aren't bathed in an unflattering harsh light. Find a large and comfortable chair, one with arms so that you may rest yours rather regally along the edges, wrists flopped over the ends. China's Dowager Empress, who reigned at the end of the nineteenth century, sat perched on an immense carved cinnabar throne. That sounds a bit cold and hard, so look for something softer to sit on. This idea sounds wacky, but think about it: Why not have one chair in your house in which you know you look impressive? Beats flopping down on an old couch when friends come to call. ⚓

withdraw often

CLOSE YOUR EYES AND DREAM WITH ME ON THIS—A ROOM OF YOUR own where you could be alone and at peace with yourself. A sanctuary. Sound unattainable? It used to be a standard feature of large houses in centuries past, and it was known as the "drawing room." It was actually a "withdrawing room," a place where ladies could gather amongst themselves and be undisturbed by the men of the house. Is there a place in your house, apartment, or maybe garden where you can carve out a withdrawing room? One determined Southern California woman built herself a tearoom in her house, from which everyone else in her family was banned. She filled it with pretty furniture positioned to take in the lovely view, added a sink and a plug-in teakettle, and always had an ample supply of fancy teas. Just the place to sit and relax with a good novel and keep the world at bay. ❧

they're playing your song

CHOOSE A THEME SONG—THINK NADIA'S THEME, NAMED FOR the young gymnast. It could be stately, like Pachelbel's Canon in D; or bittersweet, like Mozart's Piano Concerto no. 23; or a sexy, sultry jazz standard, like Shirley Horn singing "Come a Little Closer." This is something not only to listen to at night, but this is also to hear in your head as you go through the day. Select a piece of music that you can imagine playing as you enter a room. Make a tape for yourself, or buy a CD to play in your car, so that you can float through life on your own carefully chosen theme. I once had an old Mercedes in which I observed very strict rules for behavior. One rule was that I could only listen to Brazilian jazz. Imagine how it made me feel as I drove around in an otherwise ordinary suburban setting, swaying my shoulders to the sultry Brazilian jazz of Astrud Gilberto. You might pick several themes for yourself—one that you imagine playing as you stride into work every morning, one that you can hear in your head as you pull into your driveway at night, and perhaps one that you can imagine quite clearly whenever the mood for romance strikes you. ☙

old money

IMPRESSED BY THOSE ENORMOUS BANNERS AND FLAGS WITH LIONS and griffins that hang on the walls of castles, the regal emblems of a particular family or region, flapping in the breeze? But why should they have all the fun? Why not design your own family or personal crest, one that embodies the way you live your life? I did it myself a few years ago. I designed a crest that has a martini glass perched on the top of a stack of books. Gin and books—that pretty much sums up most of the folks in my family circle. What will you put on yours? An animal? A flower? Grand colors and geometric shapes? Let your imagination run wild. Once you've designed it, put it to use on napkins, stationery, or a large banner of your own to wave in the breeze. And why stop at designing a family crest? Why not also develop your own personal motto? My family's motto is "Is this my drink?" (Why do you think there is a martini glass on my family's crest?) Maybe yours will be something inspiring about strength and courage. ⚘

a place to rest your head

ONCE YOU'VE DESIGNED A FAMILY CREST OR CREATED A FAMILY motto, why not put it to use in decorating your house? Learn to needlepoint, and create a sofa full of handmade luxury pillows that are yours, and yours alone. Needlepoint is really is a mindless thing to do, not at all like knitting or crocheting, or anything else that requires you to pay attention. I create my own patterns by buying blank canvas and drawing on them with special ink pens. And then I needlepoint constantly, which has such an idle, rich-lady air to it. In addition to pillows with my "family crest" of a martini glass and books, my house is filled with needlepoint pillows with logos from favorite hotels. It is an easy thing to do, and a wonderful way to remind yourself of a special trip. Just take a pack of matches, hotel stationery, or something with the logo on it, and plop it on a copy machine turned to "enlarge." Get the logo the size you want, trace it onto blank canvas, buy thread in the colors you want, and go to it. A hundred or so hours later (I told you it was a self-indulgent way to spend time), you'll have a finished pillow. If there isn't a needlepoint store in your town, Needlepoint, Inc. of San Francisco has a very good Web site, at www.needlepointinc.com.

the woman i love

YOU KNOW THE STORY, HOW THE ENGLISH KING EDWARD VIII GAVE up his throne for "the woman I love" because she was divorced, and, as head of the Church of England, he couldn't marry her. The Duke of Windsor (the title he received after stepping down) and his Duchess never again lived in a castle, but that didn't stop

Wallis, the Duchess, from trying to replicate that feeling for her husband. She learned to run a regal house on the relatively meager sums available, and why shouldn't you, too? How did she do it? And how can you do it, too? Wallis learned a great deal from Elsie de Wolfe, one of the twentieth century's first interior designers. Elsie taught her a trick you should know—that to create a simple yet sumptuous look, all you need are mirrors on the walls, candles, and an abundance of flowers. For a really regal touch, though, type up your daily schedule. The Duke had grown accustomed to that as King, and so Wallis had it done for him always, even if it just said, "Weed flowers at 3. Have tea at 4." ↻

here's to you!

TIRED OF DRINKING OUT OF THOSE CHIPPED AND MISMATCHED wineglasses you've had since college? Put them in the back of the cupboard to use as extras, and march out and buy yourself something better. Regardless of your surroundings, you will feel elegant and cashmere-bound when balancing a nice piece of stemware in your hand. Really fancy crystal for twelve will cost a bundle; but really fancy crystal for just one or two, won't cost all that much. A wonderful place to indulge in reasonably priced crystal is at your local antique store. Won't you feel like a pampered princess when you are holding a 1920s pink crystal goblet with an art deco gold rim around the top? Those glasses were quite the rage some seventy-five years ago, and you can pick them up for $20 or so now. Raise a glass and toast yourself, my dear, for all you've done and all you have ahead of you. Cheers! ❧

come into my bedroom

I'VE TALKED ABOUT THE IMPORTANCE OF SHEETS, AND THE importance of having at least one corner of your house or apartment where things are as close to perfect and pretty as you can get. So, why not make that room your own bedroom? Even if you share it with someone else, make it an island of calm luxury. It might well be the only calm luxury you have in the house!

Redecorating your house or apartment the way you want it would cost tens of thousands of dollars. But if you can redo only one room, think about investing the money in your bedroom. Sink the money into sheets, paint the walls a flattering color, buy one of those teeny tiny sound systems that sound so good, and give yourself the gift of having one perfect room in the house. Think of the hours we all spend in our bedrooms—why would you want to spend another ten minutes in a room that doesn't reflect who you are and how you want your life to be? If you can't afford to decorate your entire bedroom, just begin with your bed and the bedside tables, so that as you sit in bed you are surrounded with the things you love. Soon enough you will be able to achieve perfection elsewhere. ❧

you look mahvelous!

I'VE SAID IT OVER AND OVER AGAIN—WE PRINCESSES DON'T wait for someone else to create an opportunity for us to indulge ourselves or our dreams, we create it ourselves. You'd love to get dressed up, but no one invites you to formal occasions? So? I hereby give you permission to put on your fanciest dress and just stay home. Not long ago I watched the David Letterman show while wearing a strapless black gown, high-heeled shoes, and a pink pashmina shawl draped over my shoulders. Just back in from a late night out on the town? No, actually. I'd put the children to bed, worked on the computer for a bit in my jeans, and then changed into a glamorous outfit just for the heck of it. I did feel like a rich and famous movie star, draped on the couch in such a grand outfit. It was a kick. Why don't you put this book down now for a few minutes, go and put on your absolutely best outfit (the one that is gathering dust in the back of your closet), and then drape yourself elegantly across the couch and keep reading? Doesn't that feel *mahvelous*? ⚓

princess school

WOULD YOU LIKE AN INSTANT COURSE IN MOVING THROUGH LIFE in a more regal manner? A living, breathing example of someone who holds her head high and moves like a princess? Then rent yourself a copy of the classic Audrey Hepburn movie *Roman Holiday*, pour yourself a glass of Italian wine or maybe a cup of espresso, and settle in to watch this great old black and white. Audrey Hepburn plays a European princess who sneaks away from her royal routine one night to experience the ordinary life. She does a wonderful job of waving the royal back-of-the-hand wave. Observe closely and try to practice the gracious nod of the head (you can use it on waiters as you order champagne before dinner), and look closely at her regal bearing. Take lessons from Audrey Hepburn's portrayal of a bored princess, and they will get you through many situations in which you feel like a fish out of water. Sort of like attending charm school from the comforts of your own couch. That's it—straight back, proud head, casual ease. Yes, you can do it, too. ◅

draped in glamour

VELVET. DOESN'T THAT WORD JUST SOUND AND FEEL LUXURIOUS when you say it? So sumptuous. Say it out loud, and feel how your lips get all pouty and sexy as you say the word. So wouldn't your world be even sexier and more sumptuous if you had velvet drapes? Deep-colored, plush velvet drapes to separate the rooms in your house—imagine what it will feel like to push one of those heavy curtains aside as you pass from room to room. Just like the tapestry hangings in old castles, velvet curtains will even help you keep your rooms toasty warm in the drafty winter months. Choose a deep, deep green or a dark red or purple for the most regal look, and fasten them back against the wall with heavy gold braided tassels. Sound expensive? It doesn't have to be, if you do it yourself with velvet remnants. And it is so much less expensive to use velvet curtains as doors in between rooms than to hang them around an entire room. Much more luxury for the buck, my dear. ⚬

red square

FOR A REGAL-LOOKING ROOM, PAINT YOUR WALLS A DEEP MAROON or red. Immediately you'll feel enveloped in glamour and intrigue. Dark walls seem to absorb the noise of our ordinary world and make us feel sealed off and protected, as though weare inside a giant shell. Although the walls in my house are, sadly, all white, as a child I spent hours in the dark red library of my parents' home. My mother was ahead of her time; she painted over the beige walls after a cousin showed slides of a trip to Communist China in the seventies. "That's it!" my mother shouted, as the edges of one photo were projected onto the wall. It was a large photo of Red Square. "That is the color I want to paint my walls!" So she did. ⚬

would you like the pink, or maybe the blue?

REMEMBER THAT, AS A PRINCESS, YOU ARE learning to speak up and ask for special things in your life. So why not speak up and ask for some help next time you go shopping? Indulge in the services of a personal shopper. Most high-end department stores have them nowadays, ready and waiting to help you find that perfect interview suit or the right outfit to wear to a fancy dinner. Like the concierges in a hotel, personal shoppers don't actually cost anything to use. They are paid by the store and are happy to help you with your needs and stay within your budget. Imagine how "with it" you will feel as you trail around a store in the wake of a personal shopper who knows just where the goodies are hidden. Why not relax and let someone else tell you what looks good on you, instead of always going for the same style and color? Who knows what you might learn? ⚓

the well-dressed table

EVEN THE MOST ORDINARY PLATES LOOK SWANK WHEN FINE LINEN napkins are lying next to them. And once again, this is the perfect lux item to pick up in an antique store instead of a department store. Think how much more impressive it will look if there are already fancy embroidered initials or monograms on them. Of course the chances that you'll find the initial of your own last name are slim, but look anyway. Heavens, perhaps you'll find a set with an actual crest! My friend Amy sells antique linens and agrees that making up a story for the unknown initial is half the fun. Tell your guests all about your eccentric imaginary ancestors. Imagine the scene: You wave your napkin casually in the air as you say, "These old things? They came from my great Uncle Bertie's house at the lake. He was a bit of a character, used to race around in an old boat waving these napkins and shouting at onlookers to get inside at once." I bought a full set of embroidered linen napkins and placemats in an antique store in Ohio for a stunning $30. It costs more to have them cleaned after a party! Start looking for yours now—you'll learn the world is full of lovely old linen. ✍

swept up in the mood

WANT TO FEEL LIKE JACKIE KENNEDY IN PARIS? OR PERHAPS A famous king's mistress? Then march straight to your hairdresser and insist on what salon ladies call an "up do." Wearing your hair "up" is guaranteed to make you feel grand as you carefully walk down the street, and you will be amazed at the difference in your attitude. The weight on your head. The exposed feeling of the back of your head. Once again, that posture will matter. And it shows off your earrings—wear really long drippy ones, please. You will feel almost naked, and very, very sexy. It makes you turn your head slowly, more regally. Jackie Kennedy liked the young Frenchman who did her hair up in a "brioche" so much that she smuggled him on the presidential press plane rather than go without his services. A word of warning: When you go to the hairdresser, don't forget to wear a shirt that buttons. Many a high-school girl has ended up in tears on prom night as her mother takes a pair of scissors to a favorite turtleneck rather than pull it over the fancy coiffure. ✿

indoor garden

LUXURIANT...SOUNDS LIKE A VARIATION ON LUXURY, DOESN'T IT? It really isn't, though it has to do with things that grow in abundance. So why not learn to create a luxuriously luxuriant indoor garden of your own, one filled with orchids? Orchids are truly the flowers that symbolize gracious living, and they also have a reputation of being difficult to grow. Only eccentric old ladies in white outfits grow orchids, don't they? Actually, orchids are not that difficult to grow, and they will give you a gorgeous growing thing to focus on in your daily life. You don't have to live in the tropics (although you can always aspire to it!) or have your own greenhouse in order to grow them. Orchids like the same kind of comfortable temperatures that your body does. Why not place an Angraecum near a window in your bathroom? It is a lovely dwarf plant that is very fragrant at night. Wouldn't that be a heavenly addition to your bath time? The smell of a delicate orchid in the air... ❧

one lump or two?

TAKING TEA—DOESN'T THAT SOUND SWANK, IN THE LAND OF Starbucks? It is, my dear, and it is an experience you should reward yourself with often. Although it actually got its start as a British working-class tradition (the tea was "high" because they perched up on stools), high tea is now a rather elegant affair served around three or four o'clock. You'll be faced with a dazzling choice of teas (my favorite is the smoky flavor of Lapsang Souchong) and an even more dazzling array of scones, thick clotted creams, tiny meaty pastries, and cute little sandwiches. Regardless of where you live, there is a high tea near you. Famous places to indulge include the Waldorf-Astoria in New York, the

Ritz-Carlton in Chicago or Boston, the Windsor Court Hotel in New Orleans, and the St. Francis Hotel in San Francisco. Wouldn't that be a self-indulgent theme to a cross-country trip— driving from one fancy tea place to the next? If you have felt unable to wear any of those swanky clothes I keep urging on you, this would be the time and place to wear them. It wouldn't be over the top to wear white gloves to tea. ↙

baby-soft

NOT EVERY LUXURIOUS MOMENT NEEDS TO INVOLVE CASHMERE, silk, candles, or champagne. Sometimes a tiny baby will do. One of life's most delicious moments is when you hold out your empty arms and cuddle a young baby. That silky soft skin, that delicious little baby smell. Mmmmm... Even if your own chil-dren have long since outgrown that little baby phase, or if you aren't a mother yourself, take advantage of every opportunity that presents itself to indulge in holding someone else's sweet baby. Wash your hands, take that baby gently in your arms, close your eyes, and drink in that wonderful smell. Nuzzle your nose in that soft warm place behind their necks, and you will remember the moment for days. ᐯ

basic black

WHAT DO YOU REALLY NEED TO GET ALONG IN LIFE? AIR, WATER, food, shelter, and some black velvet. Yes, black velvet. Along with a nice white shirt. It was sultry actress and torch singer Marlene Dietrich's basic outfit—a ruffled white blouse and black velvet pants. This go-anywhere, do-anything outfit has been reinterpreted every decade, from Twiggy in the sixties to a new Ralph Lauren variation every season. Just a few years ago, Sharon Stone caused a sensation at the Oscars when she put together a long black velvet skirt, her husband's white shirt, and a diamond-encrusted lizard pin on the back of the skirt's waistband. Now *that* is a memorable look. With black velvet pants or a black velvet skirt and a stark white shirt, you can go anywhere on a moment's notice. No need to fuss over what you are going to wear because, like the air you breathe, it is already there. ᐯ

top drawer

SPICED UNDERWEAR—DOESN'T THAT SOUND
exotic? It is, and it is also an inexpensive and
simple treat to indulge in. Earlier I mentioned
that I place scent strips from magazines in my
underwear drawer. I do, indeed. I also put fancy soaps, fresh-cut
rosemary from the garden, and even fresh herbal tea bags in my
underwear drawer—anything to give myself a nice peasant whiff
when I pull open the drawer. It is just a little private pleasure, not
one anyone else will ever be aware of. Open the drawer while getting dressed in the morning, a fairly humdrum moment in your
everyday life, but close your eyes, breathe deeply, and stay there
a moment before going on with the rest of your ordinary day. A
lovely scent on which to begin. ✿

the restful look

ALTHOUGH I HAVE JUST TRIED TO CONVINCE YOU TO PAINT AT LEAST one room in your life dark red, I'll admit that luxury doesn't always come colored in purples and reds and hung with gold swags. The famous French designer and businesswoman Coco Chanel decorated her private apartments at the Paris Ritz with the colors white, beige, and bittersweet brown. Everywhere you looked there were vases of white flowers. Doesn't that sound like a soft, subdued, and serene atmosphere in which to live? You don't have to alienate men with an overly feminine, flowery look in your home or bedroom (and Chanel never alienated any man), so chose something that will look calm and uncluttered and create an oasis of rest and ease in an otherwise busy world. ᨑ

everything in its place

LIFE ISN'T PERFECT, AND I DON'T EVER RECOMMEND TRYING TO attain perfection. I will gently point out, however, that one of the most luxurious feelings of all is to sit in the midst of a clean and uncluttered room, surveying a neat and tidy scene. It is easier to feel regal when all around you is neat and organized, and the fact is that most of us have to get it that way ourselves. As I mentioned in the introduction, children's abandoned underwear and long-forgotten Dr. Pepper cans can be found in many rooms of my house. This isn't about perfection. But I do strive to have as many moments as I can when I can look around and think—yes, it all looks under control. There is true luxury in order. ❧

a few of your favorite things

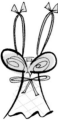 WHY SPEND THE NIGHT IN YET ANOTHER HUMDRUM
hotel room when you can relax among a few of your
own familiar objects? What princess would deign to
cross the threshold of a hotel without a few of her
favorite things? Not you. What is it that will make you
feel indulged on the road? Diana Vreeland traveled
with a "necessaire" that included a crystal carafe with brandy. I
bring along candles, framed pictures, and my favorite silk
bathrobe. Perhaps you will want to bring your own pillow or a
cozy lap blanket to throw over a hotel chair. What about fancy
bath oils that you save for traveling? A special nightgown that
makes you feel like someone other than a tired executive away
from home for yet another night? Bring something, anything, to
help remind you of how truly unique you are. ✍

a ritual existence

A LOVELY HABIT TO DEVELOP IS TO CREATE PRIVATE RITUALS FOR yourself. Moments in which you stop to drink in life's quiet beauty. Rituals in which, for just a few moments, it is simply you living the kind of life you want to live. One friend sets aside a few minutes every evening after she puts her four young children to bed. She carefully takes out a treasured china teacup—one that no one else is allowed to touch—measures out loose tea, and sits and waits patiently while it steeps. Breathing in the aroma of her own special tea helps her unwind from a busy day of teaching and mothering. Develop a small daily ritual that will make you feel less rushed, more ready to enjoy the next moment of your life. Perhaps it is spending a few minutes sitting outside every evening, looking at the stars. Or a few minutes every morning doing yoga. I had a delightful friend whose dining ritual was a wonder to behold: With a great flourish, he would fluff out a large napkin and carefully cover his ample stomach, clipping the napkin to his collar with two large gold clips that he took everywhere. Watching him prepare for a meal always gave me pleasure, because he was so clearly ready for the next moment in his life—the moment when a beautifully prepared meal would arrive. What ritual can you develop for yourself? ♠

look what you did!

THE BEST INDULGENCES AND LUXURIES DON'T ALWAYS REQUIRE A monetary investment. Consider the luxury of being able to cheer yourself up whenever you need it. How is that possible? Simple. I want you to take out a fresh piece of paper and begin to list in great detail every little thing you have accomplished in life. Give yourself credit for *everything*, even seemingly small things like your ability to make the grumpy grocery store checker smile. Before Letitia Baldridge was Jackie Kennedy's social secretary, she worked at Tiffany & Company and didn't get quite the positive feedback she'd hoped for from an employer. "After my first year at Tiffany's, I decided that what I needed to do to keep from being totally depressed was to make a written list of my sizable accomplishments...and go over it repeatedly in my mind while everyone else in the store was yelling at me. My own philosophy kept me afloat." What a grand idea! Imagine how much better you will feel when a low moment hits you, if you can just duck into a private area, pull out your carefully compiled list, and indulge in a quick pat on the back, an "attagirl" moment for yourself. As a matter of fact, why wait until you are feeling low? ⚘

breakfast (and a bath) at tiffany's

I HOPE YOU AREN'T FEELING LEFT OUT WHEN I TOSS AROUND THE big names of luxury such as Tiffany & Company, or prattle on about expensive things like cashmere. Because the fact is, you really should treat yourself at least once in your young life to a little something from Tiffany's. Now, it needn't cost very much; I don't want you to overspend. There are plenty of inexpensive things you can buy at Tiffany & Company, from scented soaps

($35) to a small cut-crystal bowl ($30). The sight of
that famous blue shopping bag or wrapping paper is a
guaranteed thrill. I have found a wonderful way to
keep the luxury of the Tiffany's label around me for free—I save
the little shopping bags from my meager purchases and use them
as swank-looking flower vases around the house. How? I just
pour water into a small drinking glass, set it down inside the
shopping bag, and plop cut flowers into the glass, letting them
drape over the sides of the bag. A very posh look. ❧

creamy bliss

A DELICIOUS INDULGENCE YOU MUST LEARN TO MAKE IS LOBSTER
bisque, a creamy and richly flavored soup to savor on any occasion. And once you can make lobster bisque, you can learn to
make crab bisque, or tomato bisque, or any one of a number of
rich and creamy soups. Do you sense a theme here to the few
recipes that I insist you master and add to your culinary reper-
toire? Thick, creamy, luscious, and well...rich. Very rich.

Lobster bisque is the soup version of "chocolate cashmere," as I christened the homemade chocolate pudding.

Lobster Bisque from The Silver Palate Good Times Cookbook

2 gallons water
2 live lobsters (1 to 1 1/4 pounds each)
6 tablespoons (3/4 stick) butter
1/3 cup cognac
1/2 cup plus 3 tablespoons chopped shallots
2 cloves garlic, minced
3 tablespoons tomato paste
2 1/2 cups dry white wine
1 teaspoon dried tarragon
1/2 teaspoon dried thyme
pinch red pepper flakes
2 bay leaves
3 tablespoons unbleached all-purpose flour
2 1/2 cups milk
3/4 cup heavy or whipping cream
salt and freshly ground black pepper, to taste
2 egg yolks

1. In a large stockpot, heat the water to boiling. Drop in the lobsters and cook, covered, for 12 minutes. Remove the lobsters from the pot; reserve 4 cups of the water. Let the lobsters cool.

2. When the lobsters are cool enough to handle, crack the shells and remove all the lobster meat. Finely dice the meat and set aside. Reserve the shells.

3. In a large skillet, melt half the butter over medium heat. Add the lobster shells and pour in the cognac. Heat until the cognac is warm, then flame it with a match. When the flames subside, stir in 1/2 cup of the shallots, the garlic, tomato paste,

wine, reserved cooking liquid, tarragon, thyme, red pepper flakes, and bay leaves. Simmer, uncovered, for 30 minutes. Strain through a sieve into a bowl.

4. In a stockpot, over medium-high heat, melt the remaining 3 tablespoons of butter. Add the reamining 3 tablespoons of shallots and sauté for 2 minutes. Add the flour and cook, whisking constantly, for 1 minute. Gradually whisk in the strained lobster stock; whisk until well blended. Whisk in the milk and cream, then heat over medium heat until hot. Season to taste with salt and pepper.

5. Whisk the egg yolks together in a small bowl. Whisk in $1/2$ cup of the hot soup, then return to the pot; whisk until thoroughly blended. Stir in the reserved lobster meat. Heat for several minutes and serve immediately. Serves 6 quite nicely. ᴧ

who's that girl?

YOU'VE SEEN THE PICTURES. JACKIE O IN A T-SHIRT AND JEANS, hiding behind those huge round dark glasses as she strides down the road in Capri. Even if she wasn't the most famous woman in the world back then, you'd wonder who she was. So why not make people wonder who *you* are? Indulge in the biggest and blackest-lensed pair of sunglasses you can lay your dainty hands on, and get out there on the public stage. The great thing about sunglasses is that they are an inexpensive way to indulge in very pricey designer names. Chanel, Prada, Versace—you name the fashion house, they've got a pair of sunglasses to sell you at a price far less than that of anything else they make! It might cost thousands for a piece of clothing with that label, but just $100 or so for the fanciest sunglasses. Once you've got your hands on your big glamour glasses, you might want to try pairing them with your silk scarf for yet another movie-star-in-hiding sort of look. ⚘

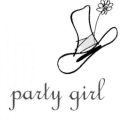

party girl

NOW IT IS TIME TO PUT THESE RICH AND DELICIOUS RECIPES TO work and become a skilled hostess, to indulge your friends and family, and to be indulged in turn . Guests will soon learn that you don't serve skimpy salads. One of the few times I've left a lunch hungry was after a limp and tiny offering of salad at the California Governor's house one hot afternoon. Make sure your guests leave savoring the last rich tastes of your bisque on their lips, your chocolate pudding on their shirt fronts. Famed Washington D.C. hostess Sally Quinn says that the best parties must have a theme; your guests should always know what the point of your party is. And Pat Montandon, a well-known San Francisco socialite and the author of a seventies book called *How to Be a Party Girl*, believes that you should gather up the most interesting people you know and sit them down at a table to see what will happen. She held a series of Round Table luncheons for years, sending out invitations to names in the news and fascinating folks she'd just met. Mix them all up together, and there you have it. Whom can you invite to create your own interesting social melange? ♨

national velvet

ADMIT IT, YOU LOVED HORSES WHEN YOU WERE A GIRL, DIDN'T you? Most women did. Entire psychology books have been devoted to why women like horses. I have my own theory: It's the clothes. You've seen those grand-looking women at the scene of an English hunt, dressed in such elegant attire. Who wouldn't want to be able to walk around like that in ordinary life? So go ahead and recapture a bit of your girlish youth, while at the same time including some luxury in your life—put down this book and sign up for riding lessons. (I mean English, of course. Sexy as cowboys look on their Western saddles, it just isn't as elegant as those sleek and spare English saddles.) Riding lessons also help you improve your posture and bearing, and they have an additional bonus: Riding horses tightens your thighs! And then there is the wardrobe—leather riding boots, tight-fitting jodhpurs, and a smart-looking black velvet helmet. ⚓

dining al fresco

FEEL THE BREEZE ON YOUR FACE, THE SOFT GRASS UNDER you. Such a lovely scene: You and a friend at an outdoor picnic, reclining on a blanket and sipping out of long-stem glasses. Pity there isn't a string quartet nearby to provide a lush sound, but we can't have everything, can we? The self-indulgent girl has her picnic set all ready to go, on a moment's notice, for these impromptu occasions: a nice thick blanket or quilt, a nice big straw basket, linen napkins. Pull together some of the other tiny luxuries that you now have—a few good glasses, a china plate or two, and those monogrammed linen napkins. Buying an already put together picnic hamper doesn't cost much nowadays, less than $100 for a straw suitcase fitted with everything you need, including the tiny salt and pepper shakers. What are you waiting for? Go outdoors and eat. ᐱ

let the sun shine

WHILE YOU ARE DEVELOPING THE HABIT OF DINING OUTSIDE WITH your new picnic things, here is another old-fashioned habit I'd encourage you to indulge in. Close your eyes, turn your face to the sun, and relax for a few minutes in the warmth. What? Without sunscreen? Gasp, that seems so shockingly daring nowadays. The fact is, the newest research shows that we are actually beginning to suffer a bit from the effects of not letting sun shine on our skin! Our bodies need sun to create vitamin D, which keeps our bones strong and healthy. Why not indulge in a face full of sunshine every so often, skin wrinkles be damned. I'm not suggesting you lie out unprotected all afternoon while your picnic wilts beside you, but do give yourself a chance to soak up a bit of sun before you pull the sunscreen out of the bag. ⚘

signature gift

 DEVELOP A REPUTATION FOR GIVING THE SAME thoughtful present over and over and over...Some folks bring along their homemade mustards or jams. Paul Newman's hostess gift of homemade salad dressing grew into the Newman's Own company. In the Kennedy White House, Jackie developed a signature gift of a paperweight of a large, uncut semiprecious stone, such as malachite or rose quartz, taken from U.S. soil, wrapped like a parcel in eighteen-karat gold rope by a jeweler, and put on a small base with an engraved message. A bit grand for the rest of us, but you can achieve the same thing by always showing up with an armload of fresh-cut flowers or herbs from your garden, or a loaf of fresh-baked bread. My signature wedding gift is an old book published in the forties called *I Married Adventure*, by Osa Johnson. I hunt them down in used bookstores around the country. The cover has a wonderful zebra-skin design, and the title makes a memorable slogan for any marriage. And I get a great thank-you card every time! Develop a signature gift-wrap look, too, one that your friends will always recognize. So what will *your* signature be? ₰

moon garden

IMAGINE A PLACE WHERE YOU COULD SIT UNDER THE STARS AND breath in the smells of exotic night-blooming flowers. Why not make a moon garden of your very own? Fill planters or pots around a patio with night-blooming jasmine, tuberoses, honeysuckle, the moonflower type of morning glory, or—best of all— night phlox, which is also known as "midnight candy" for its sticky sweet scent. Indulge your senses, close your eyes, and feel the cool evening air kiss your skin. For another otherworldly touch, put garden candles all around the edges of the patio to make your own fairy palace in the forest, your very own garden of romance and relaxation. Sleep outside to truly indulge in the wonder of the night sky, the cool air, and the floral scents. ₰

the vintage look

AS A GIRL , I HAD SUCH A LONGING FOR A LARGE FUR COAT. I THINK
it came from a scene in Dr. Zhivago, where one of the actresses
is swathed in white fur and riding in the back of a horse-drawn
sleigh. So enchanting. For the price of a fur you can buy a
small car, though, so how can you get a tiny bit of that glamour
into your life without having to take the bus? The answer is:
vintage. I am the delighted owner of a vintage curly black Persian
lamb coat from the forties, and my friends exclaim with delight
whenever I show up wearing it. The price of a car? No, the price
of a Greyhound bus ticket. I paid $75 for it. Type in "vintage fur"
on eBay and see what delightful things come up. Perhaps you'll
find old cashmere sweaters with lush fur collars, just the thing to
add to your new standard outfit of black velvet pants and a crisp
white shirt. ❧

a bit of cheer

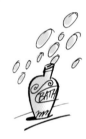

LIFE IS FULL OF WONDERFUL SLOGANS AND BITS OF INSPIRATIONAL writing. Why not choose your favorite, print it up nicely on your computer, and then put it in a fancy frame to be prominently displayed in a place where it will give you strength whenever you need it? Around my house you can take strength from the words of Winston Churchill, framed and perched next to the sink: *Winston Churchill's Recipe for a Happy Life—Hot baths, cold champagne, new peas, and old brandy.* Or next to my bar you'll find this bit of inspiration from Robert Benchley, a member of the old Algonquin Hotel Round Table set: *Get me out of this wet coat and into a dry martini!* Any words look important when encased in a fancy frame. Choose your words and frame them.

small, but perfect

ANOTHER SMALL ROOM IN WHICH TO INDULGE YOURSELF ON A budget is your very own bathroom. Giving your bathroom a luxurious gloss is even less of a budget drain than redoing a bedroom, and once again it gives you one tiny perfect world in which you can cloister yourself. Imagine the perfect world of luxury you can create in a few hundred square feet for just a few hundred dollars! Fresh scented flowers and candles go a long way in a small room, too. You can have fun with the color of your bathroom, and perhaps change the lighting to give it an enchanted look. My own favorite room in my house is the guest bathroom, where the wallpaper looks like book endpapers, and I've adorned the walls with an assortment of old political mementos, old maps, and other quaint things I've found over the years at garage sales and antique stores. It looks a bit like an English men's club, and my guests feel like visiting dignitaries. Add an expensive hand towel, and the look is pure luxury for a tiny, tiny sum. ⟨⟩

for your eyes only

WHY NOT INDULGE YOURSELF IN SOME PRIVATE WAY THAT ONLY
you will know? Being secretly indulged is a marvelous feeling.
You can be secretly indulged under your clothes (knowing that
underneath your ordinary boots and blue jeans, your toes are
wearing cashmere socks), or even inside your own mind. Be
secretly indulged mentally by having peace of mind, one un-
burdened by worries and concerns. Perhaps you can secretly
enjoy the knowledge that you have assets (and I do want you to
build them!), or the luxury of a financial security, knowing you
are not burdened by debts. What about the luxury to say NO?
Arriving at a place in your life and in your self-confidence
where you can pleasantly say "no" to someone is a tremendous
luxury. ❧

at your service

OH LOOK, THE BUTLER IS HERE WITH OUR DRINKS! OH, maybe not. You can easily make it look as if the butler has just been here, though. All it takes is a nice drinks tray to set out on the table. Just that one little gesture makes the simple act of bringing a drink to someone look quite grand and posh. Drinks trays are everywhere in the stores; you can spend a little or you can spend a lot. I spent a little and then made it look as if I spent a lot...by starting with a cheap wooden $10 tray. I painted it a deep maroon color, then cut up all of those swanky magazine ads I mentioned earlier. My tray is decorated with tiny diamonds, large glossy pearls, and Ralph Lauren outfits. Cut up the look you want, glue the pieces in place, and apply a decoupage layer to make it waterproof. ❧

the lavender effect

SLIDE UNDER YOUR SHEETS AND TAKE A LONG, DEEP BREATH. WHAT is that marvelous smell? Could it be that you've just spritzed your sheets with lavender sheet spray? Lavender, in addition to its wonderful fragrance, is also an herb long reputed to help you fall asleep at night. Who wouldn't want to be enveloped in such a heady smell while floating gently off to sleep? I've found that the best (and one of the least expensive) of the lavender sheet sprays comes from The Good Home Company and sells for around $16. You can find it on their Web site at www.goodhomeco.com. You could also enjoy the same effect by leaving a lavender sachet on your pillow during the daytime and removing it at night (too lumpy and scratchy!). Make your own sachet by drying lavender sprigs and then collecting the buds to sew into a little pouch. ❧

her highness on the road

TRAVEL USED TO BE VIEWED AS A LUXURY, BUT THOSE DAYS ARE long gone. Airline travel hardly seems like a luxurious experience anymore, but there are several ways in which your inner princess can be indulged on the road. To travel like a princess, you can do several things: Bring your own favorite foods to eat on the plane, seek out quiet spots in airports where you can relax (such as the big white rocking chairs at La Guardia), carry a warm shawl to tuck around you in the chill of the plane, and best of all—don't carry any luggage. Either travel as light as possible or ship your luggage ahead via some other method. You want to be striding unencumbered through the airport, not schlepping heavy bags. Remember to bring toasty warm socks to slip on during the flight after you've removed your shoes. If you are really feeling princess-like and ready to be indulged on the road, get a massage. In many airports now you'll find mini-spas with ten-minute massage services. A delicious treat for $20!

her highness at work

TENSE AND TIRED AT WORK? ONCE AGAIN ANNOYED WITH THE coworker who keeps shirking his duties? Wouldn't you love to leave this scene behind and be at a spa right now? Alas, most of us do have to work, but there are ways that we can be indulged at the office on a regular basis. Build yourself a desk-spa to keep in a drawer at work. Include a massage ball for your back and feet, peppermint foot lotion or spray, a face spritzer, and some heavy, rich hand cream. Close your door for a few minutes and relax. For those cube-dwelling princesses, just put a few of these things in your purse, walk down the hall, and hide in a bathroom stall to indulge yourself. It might not be the most elegant of surroundings, but it will certainly do the trick. Just think how much easier it will be to face the rest of the day once you've spent even a few minutes alone with scented lotion and a quick self-massage. Master a few mini-yoga moves that you can do at your desk, and let the calmness wash over you. ❧

not the wrong fork

OSCAR WILDE ONCE FAMOUSLY SAID, "THE WORLD WAS MY oyster, but I used the wrong fork!" Why feel frantic and nervous in social situations when, with just a little study, you can be relaxed and at ease? Being confident of your social skills is a great way to be "secretly indulged." The posh magazine *Town & Country* gathered up their "Social Graces" columns and published them in a book by the same name. You might not need the etiquette lesson about how to properly thank the owner of the private plane you've just flown in, but the other essays about gossip, cell phone use, and proper restaurant behavior are a bit more practical. As a child, I had a book called *White Gloves and Party Manners*, which was filled with information about how to properly introduce two people (introduce the younger person to the older person, as a sign of respect) and how to behave at the table. It is still in print after all these years, and you are never too old to brush up on these social skills. And then, you can relax. ❧

here's to you!

PERHAPS YOU'VE BEGUN TO SENSE A THEME IN ALL OF THESE ideas—don't wait for someone else to send flowers, don't wait to dress up or pull out the good china. And don't wait for a special occasion to buy a good bottle of wine and drink it yourself. *You* are the special occasion, my dear. Life is special, and so are you. If you read about an interesting type of wine in a review, don't file it away for future use the next time you have guests over. March out to the store and find yourself a bottle. Wine stores can be intimidating, so just smile and ask for help. Ask the salesfolk to recommend a good bottle of wine for, say, "someone in a good mood." Or perhaps get a recommendation for an appropriate wine to drink on a Wednesday. You will get a smile back from them, guaranteed. If you do decide to indulge yourself with a special bottle of wine, please spread it over several nights. It is hard to feel like a princess with a throbbing head and a bubbly tummy. ⚘

a job for professionals

SOMETIMES THE BEST THINGS IN LIFE REALLY ARE free, such as the chance to have a professional makeup artist do your face at a department store makeup counter. Sure, they do it because they hope you will immediately buy all of the lovely products they have just applied to your face, but there is generally no obligation. I once arrived early for a business dinner in the Silicon Valley during the dot-com boom days. Instead of gulping down an espresso and reading a techie magazine to kill time like the rest of the go-getters, I plopped down in a chair at the Bobbi Brown counter at Neiman Marcus. Forty-five minutes later I emerged back into the venture capital fray, relaxed and looking spectacular, for the price of a tube of moisturizer. I haven't looked that good since! Working up the nerve to sit in the chair at one of these counters can be difficult; professional makeup artists can be as intimidating as...wine salesmen. But once you take the plunge and get over your fear, you will be delighted. This is always a fine time to try out a new look. Some women take advantage of this service whenever they have a big event scheduled. This might work for you, too, but I'd advise against trying any kind of a wild new look before a special night out. ☙

the island of calm

THE TYRANNY OF THE CELL PHONE, PAGER, AND INSTANT MESSAGES makes us all available 24/7. But why not decide *not* to be available? Whether it is just one night a week, or every night after 8 P.M., just take a stand and unplug it all. Create the luxury of silence, the thrill of being out of touch, shipwrecked on your own desert island of calm. Be mysterious, unavailable, unapproachable sometimes. There is no reason we should be available to all people at all times, and your friends and family may well secretly admire you when you announce that, henceforth (a good princess-sounding term), you will not be taking calls on Thursdays. That is the day, you tell all who will listen, that you are reserving for yourself. It will be hard to convince others to leave you alone, but if you stick to your guns you could actually start a trend! ⟨⟨

slow down

"HURRY! HURRY UP! WE'VE GOT TO GO!" HOW OFTEN DO YOU hear yourself saying *that*? Wouldn't it be a tremendous luxury to just stop, take a deep breath, and slow down your life for a while? So much of what makes us rush is really artificial. Will the world end if we arrive three minutes later at our destination? Wouldn't our day be more enjoyable if we started it off in a leisurely manner? Why not decide to wake up an hour earlier, long before anyone else in your household, so that you can sit in the garden and read the newspaper with a hot cup of coffee? Or leave the house with plenty of time to spare, so that you can enjoy your drive, knowing that you've built extra time into your schedule and can perhaps stop off at that cute little café you always have to drive by in such a rush every morning. Our lives in America are famously rushed. A European movement called Slow Food is gaining popularity on our shores. One of the major beliefs of the Slow Food folks is that we must relax and enjoy the moment around the dinner table. Slow down and savor everything before you: food, time, friends, family. You will enjoy it all so much more, and the memories will be that much sharper. 🐦

would you please?

"THE RICH ARE DIFFERENT," F. SCOTT FITZGERALD famously said. Although Hemingway's snide retort was that the rich were different because they had more money, I say it has to do with staff. The rich have people who do things for them. Big things and little things, many of life's little annoyances are swept away by someone else, leaving the rich to relax and have a nice time. Wouldn't it be nice to have your own staff? Well, in some ways you can nowadays. For centuries, hotels have had the position of "concierge," someone on the hotel staff who is always available to help guests with minor (or major!) requests. When traveling, you should certainly make it a habit to use the hotel concierge to help make arrangements during your stay; most large hotels have them. Dinner reservations, driving instructions, shopping suggestions, they know it all! Concierges have now spread beyond hotels, however, and can also be found in some big office buildings and shopping malls. A hotel concierge's services are free to guests, while the concierges working elsewhere will probably charge a small fee. But wouldn't it be worth it to have "staff" helping you smooth over some of life's bumps, however briefly? ❧

all wrapped up

WONDERFUL AS IT IS TO EMERGE SPARKLING CLEAN FROM A BATH or shower, there is always that awkward moment when, after being enveloped in the warmth of the water, you encounter the chill as you step out. Warm towels are the answer, my dear. Warm and fluffy towels to wrap yourself in and relish the feeling of being cocooned in plush cotton. The British have long had in their bathrooms strange contraptions of pipes and water on which to drape and warm your towels. They are also available in this country in many bath stores, but a budget-minded princess could do something else. Pop your towels into the dryer while you shower, so that you can instantly wrap yourself in that toasty goodness. To indulge your skin as well as your body, slather on lots of lotion and wrap up for a few minutes to let the extra warmth give you a silky smoothness. ❧

the prince of wales

IN HONOLULU I CONFIDENTLY ORDER A PRINCE OF WALES FROM the bartender. And then when they look puzzled, I tell them how to make it: light rum, dark rum, and club soda. "That is what Walter Dillingham of Honolulu served the Prince of Wales, in the twenties, when he came to call. It was the only liquor he had in the house, you see, so he mixed it up into a new drink and named it after his guest," I tell them, teaching them a tiny bit of little-known Hawaiian history. How wonderful to have your own private drink, named after you! So, why not invent one for yourself?

Mix together your favorite kinds of alcohol, name it, and start to serve it to your friends. If a drink seems too technical, why not invent a signature dish? Many famous dishes are named after actual people, from Beef Stroganoff to Peach Melba. I always serve my guests a dish I call Granite Bay Cassoulet, a streamlined variation on the traditional French cassoulet (it varies in that it takes only two days to prepare, instead of three). Imagine how immortal you will feel once you begin naming your food and drink. ↬

but my friends call me bitsy

SOMETIMES OUR ORDINARY, EVERYDAY LIVES JUST SEEM SO, WELL, ordinary and everyday. Why not step out of that life ever so briefly by creating a second one? Do you really think "Gin" Sander is my real name? No, I decided when I was forty that I wanted to rename myself with a more dashing image. Gin Sander isn't driving children to school in the morning or running a load of laundry. Gin Sander is trying to decide which hotel in Paris has a better view of Notre Dame at night, or whether to downhill or cross-country ski later this afternoon. I give out the name when I make dinner reservations, so that I really feel like a different person stepping out at night, leaving my ordinary mommy personality at home. Why not choose the name you've always wanted, and start using it on odd occasions? Not for fraudulent reasons, mind you, just as a way to allow yourself a moment to live a slightly more dashing life. Perhaps you want to create a personality based on one of your glamour role models or an elegant woman from history. Practice saying it—isn't it fun to think of yourself as someone other than who you've always been?

plush upholstery

BECOME ACQUAINTED—AND AT EASE—WITH THE LOBBIES OF grand hotels. Why buy a room for hundreds of dollars a night when you can sink down into a velvet couch and relax for an hour or two? As I write this, I am rocking gently in a comfortable rocking chair on the wide front porch of Waikiki Beach's oldest luxury hotel, the Moana Surfrider. I am not, however, a guest at this hotel. I'm staying much farther down the beach at a bargain affair. But I look so relaxed and such a part of things here in the lobby, who would question me? Even if you can't afford to stay at an expensive hotel, you can sink into a soft cushy chair for a cocktail. Just sail right in as if you belong there, never giving them the chance to question whether you do. True confession—while having a drink at a hotel bar I do swipe an extra cocktail napkin or two to use at my own bar at home. It looks quite posh to your guests at home. Find yourself a hotel that you aspire to, and begin to settle in. Absorb the quiet hum of a well-run organization, learn from the well-heeled guests. Sit there well-dressed and confident, and you will not be asked to leave. My philosophy has long been this: Act as if you own the world, and perhaps someday you will.

THE MARBLE PALACE

The most beautiful bathroom in all of California is at a hotel and restaurant complex called the Harris Ranch, midway between Sacramento and Los Angeles. Fabulous Spanish tile. I'm always in such a rush to finish up this long trip that I hardly ever eat there, and I've only once spent the night, but I certainly do stop and make myself at home in their bathroom. An indulgence tip to you all: Always use the bathroom in the best hotels. The more acquainted you become with the bars in hotel lobbies, the easier it will be for you to feel at home using their facilities whenever the mood strikes. ॐ

red meat, red wine, dark chocolate

YES, YOU READ THAT CORRECTLY: RED MEAT, RED WINE, AND DARK chocolate. I firmly believe that these are important food groups. Self-indulgent, to be sure, but important nevertheless. On a regular basis you should relax your rigid adherence to whatever diet regime you strictly adhere to, and construct a meal around these delicious three. Imagine this: The heavenly scent of a prime rib roast in your oven, the ruby-red sheen of a glass of Cabernet in your hand, and the knowledge that a chocolate tart awaits you at the end of the meal. Need I go on? Design a dinner party around this theme, and indulge your friends. On occasion I invite women over for my Red Wine and Black Dresses parties (you'll learn about those in a minute!), and as you can imagine, I get the rest of the menu from the red meat and dark chocolate food groups. Since we look like a group of nuns in our solemn dark party dresses, we've christened ourselves the Devout Sisters of the Vine. Please feel free to borrow this moniker and invite your friends to join you in your own group! ৵

puttin' on the tux

MEN ALWAYS FUSS ABOUT DRESSING UP, YET THEY LOOK SO DELICIOUS in tuxedos. So why not skip hearing them fuss, and wear a tuxedo yourself? You are certain to look delicious, too, and feel like a sexy woman of mystery and intrigue. How can you find a men's tux that fits? Well, you probably won't. Every so often a designer such as Yves St. Laurent or Ralph Lauren will come out with a high-priced tux outfit for women, but I think a better bet is to find yourself an oversized vintage tuxedo in a resale shop and take it to a tailor. Have it cut down to fit your own curves perfectly, and accessorize to your heart's content. Don't stop at the tuxedo itself; find some elegant cufflinks to wear and a jazzy silk cumberbund to wrap tightly around your waist. Perhaps wear a flouncy skirt to make the outfit more feminine looking. ৵

a house with history

EVER HEARD OF CHATSWORTH, CLIVEDEN, OR GREY GARDENS?
What about Highgrove Farm or Balmoral? They are all famous
houses. Why shouldn't a princess like yourself also live in a house
with a name? I live in a Craftsman-style bungalow house called
Shingle Belle; my family's summer house in Washington is called
Century Farm. Are these enormous houses with a long associa-
tion with the name? Not really. But don't they sound that way?
What should you call your place? You can name it after the style
of architecture, or the natural setting, or even your favorite
color. Be creative—name it, no matter how humble, and you will
feel as if your digs are super swanky. Why not invite new friends
over to your apartment, The Pillow Palace? Or maybe your
house, Dahlia Cottage? Of course it is pretentious, but so are
many fun things in life. ⚓

please join me

 NOW THAT YOU HAVE YOUR OWN TUXEDO, A BLACK velvet skirt, elegant personalized stationery, and you know how to make several delicious rich dishes, you are ready to step into the world of luxury entertaining. Put your clothes and your skills together, and invite your stylish women friends (remember, men just fuss about dressing up, and it puts such a damper on things) to your newly named abode for a Red Wine and Black Dresses party. Or create your own theme. Perhaps an annual 29th birthday party for all and sundry to enjoy? Or a party to celebrate the arrival of spring tulips and daffodils in your yard? Whatever the theme, you will be confident, relaxed, and ready to share your new attitude of indulgence and luxury with your friends. Rest assured, they will join you in your new attitude! And before you know it, you will be hosting—or getting invited to—countless lovely occasions that you will enjoy. See, why wait for something to happen in your life? Make it happen yourself! ⁣↝

travel through time

WANT TO SPEND THE DAY REALLY DRESSED LIKE A REGAL PRINCESS, enjoying the courtly bows and nods from passing gentlemen? Then make haste, my lady, to a Renaissance Faire. These fairs imaginatively reenact a period in history that you will slip into easily, a period when women were draped in sensuous velvet dresses and laced tightly into sexy bustiers. Don't have a Renaissance-period dress already hanging in your closet? No need to despair, as most of the Renaissance Faires held around the country have big booths near the entrance that will rent you a princess outfit for the day. As you walk among the crowds dressed in your luxurious finery, you will also get the chance to admire men in tight pants wearing swords and leather jerkins. Does sound like fun, doesn't it? There are large groups of people who aren't content to do this just once a year at the Faires, but have instead formed the Society for Creative Anachronism in order to play-act their Lord and Lady fantasies year-round.

There are many small regional fairs, but the biggest are in New York; Southern and Northern California; and Bristol, Wisconsin. Check it out at www.Renfair.com. ◆

from the collection of...

INTERESTED IN ACQUIRING A LUXURIOUS HABIT? LUXURIOUS, BUT not necessarily expensive? Why not form a collection of something? Start collecting items such as ceramic rabbits, or hand-blown glass Christmas ornaments, or some such thing. Collecting can take you all over the world and allow you to meet fascinating people. Once you decide what theme and what kinds of things you want to collect, you can plan trips around it, join clubs, and create events around your collection. Whether it is antique scarves, or eighteenth-century china *objets*, collecting (with all of its arcane knowledge) makes for great party chatter. "What do you collect?" you'll be able to ask people, and once they share their long story of finding the perfect Danish Christmas plate, you'll be able to regale them with stories of your own interesting things. And then you can get your friends and family interested, too. My husband is the fourth generation in his family to collect art pottery—imagine the collection he inherited and what he can pass on to our sons. Personally, I collect Chanel pearl jewelry, which sounds far posher than it really is (most Chanel is costume jewelry, you know, or *faux* as we say in French!). And I sometimes give them as gifts in the hope that it will inspire someone else to begin collecting as well. Another lovely bonus is that when you turn your attentions to your hobby, it can lead you into your own private world for a few hours, tuning out the chaos of the world while you dust and arrange your pretty little things and plan your next collecting foray in search of some elusive item. ❧

warm rinse

EACH ONE OF US HAS HER OWN FAVORITE WAY OF FEELING indulged. For some, it is buying an expensive item; for others, a quiet hour to themselves. In this book I've tried to expand your ideas about other things you can try. When I asked my own masseuse what she thinks is self-indulgent, she hesitated not a whit before telling me: *To lie back and have someone else wash my hair.* I agree. The combination of head massage, aromatherapy from the lovely shampoo, and warm water relaxation—what could be better? Well, it could be better if someone came to your house every morning and you could lie back in a soft velvet chair and be indulged. Failing that, having a loving partner do this in the shower, tub, or even sink is still delicious. Try it. Close your eyes and enjoy the sensation of his or her nails lightly tickling your skin, the foamy lather working its way into your tired scalp, and the incredible sensation of pulsing warm water pouring over your tipped-back head. Ahhh...

speak up

SOMETIMES THE GREATEST LUXURY OF ALL IS SPEAKING YOUR MIND and freely expressing your opinions. Get over being afraid of what other folks will think of you. To heck with them. Be honest about what you feel. I understand that you might not be able to do this at home or at work, so why not indulge in speaking your mind somewhere else, such as in a restaurant? "And how is your steak?" the unctuous waiter says in passing. Don't be afraid to tell him it tastes like leather and you want another one brought round immediately. Somerset Maugham once said something that I believe is quite true: "It's a funny thing about life; if you refuse to accept anything but the best, you very often get it." ⁂

late-night indulgence

YEARING FOR A CHANCE TO ENTER SOME OF YOUR CITY'S finer dining establishments, but not sure if you can afford the price of a meal? Hey, who needs a meal? Why not just go out late at night for dessert? It is usually the cheapest item on the menu, and makes for an easy way to indulge at fancy places. Why not make the whole excursion an occasion, and get as dressed up for dessert as you would for a fancy meal? Or even dressier? Think about this: If you show up at a swanky restaurant in the evening, dressed in formal attire, all the other guests will wonder what fab party you attended that they weren't invited to. This will be even more mysterious if it is midweek. And never doubt that you will be

 welcomed. Restaurant hearts gladden at the sight of well-dressed patrons arriving, as it adds a bit of gloss to the scene. As I write this, the taste of a piece of lemon cheesecake with a pine-nut crust still lingers in my mouth, and it was a Wednesday night. Heads did turn a bit as I entered in a vintage black crepe dress, but that only added to the fun! ❧

what would jackie do?

IN THE PRECEDING PAGES, I'VE INTRODUCED YOU TO (OR PERHAPS just reminded you of) a number of my self-indulgence idols—Diana Vreeland, Coco Chanel, and Wallis Windsor, to name a few. There are moments in my life when I stop and think, "How would Coco handle this?" Or, "What would Jackie do?" To heck with who I think is worth modeling, why not choose a style icon of your own? It might be a glamorous figure from the past, or perhaps your style icon won't be a name others would recognize. It could be a real live person that you know and admire for the certain something she possesses. Could it be a stylish and learned woman in your own community? My Auntie Bee, a stylish woman who lives in Carmel, California, frequently reminds me of the two big icons in her life, Phebe and Nina. Two cousins born at the turn of the last century, these incredible women did loom large in Bee's life and in mine. How amazing it was to see the verve and beauty they brought to their daily lives, from the drapes they chose (Nina used purple shower curtains in her living room) to the way they spoke (Nina again, who in her late eighties, after eating a piece of lemon meringue pie, said, "If I ever ask to eat that again, just have me killed instead."). Is there someone like that you've overlooked in your life? Seek her out and sit at her feet to learn. A style icon worth considering is Letitia Baldridge, the author of the book *A Lady, First*. She writes of her life in the American Embassy in Paris, the Kennedy White House, and the headquarters of Tiffany & Company. How could you *not* learn from her? ❧

room service

YOU KNOW HOW TO MAKE YOUR BED. WHO DOESN'T? BUT DO YOU know how to make your bed look like the bed in a four-star Asian hotel? I'm not talking about a mint on your pillow, either. I'm talking about using three sheets. "Three sheets of pure Irish linen," says my dear friend Betty Lou Dillingham, who knows a thing or two about Asian hotels. Here is what you do: Go ahead and make your bed the way you usually would, with a fitted sheet, a flat top sheet, and a blanket or two. But then...you take out yet another flat sheet, and you smooth it sharply across the blankets. Turn back the original top sheet over the top, near your pillows, tuck the whole thing in tightly, and there you have it. It looks neat and luxurious, and trust me—it feels wonderful. No more scratchy blankets near your chin, just acres of smooth cotton to stroke you at night. If you take extra time in the morning to make your bed perfectly, it will look like a posh hotel when you come in at night. Now if only you could get someone to come in every evening and do the thing with the chocolates, wouldn't life be a dream? ⬥

home spa day

I DON'T HAVE TO TELL YOU THAT A FULL DAY AT A SPA IS TOTALLY self-indulgent and luxurious. I also don't have to tell you that it is expensive! What isn't particularly expensive for girls like us, though, is to set aside one day a month to indulge in a spa day at home. All it requires is a trip to the grocery store. I admit it is hard to feel pampered and glamorous while cruising the aisles at the A&P picking up supplies for your spa day, but do the best you can. What should you put in your grocery cart? How about this: olive oil, a can of tomato paste, a basket of fresh strawberries, and several lemons. Is this a pasta recipe? No. Here is what you do: Pour a half cup or so of the olive oil into a mug and warm it ever so slightly in the microwave. Using your fingers, work it into the ends of your hair. Pin your hair up, and leave the oil in for at least half an hour. (When shampooing, apply the shampoo to dry hair and work it in, then lather it up. That helps soak up the extra oil.) Wash and dry your face, and then either use smashed strawberries as a fresh fruit facial or just slather on tomato paste straight from the can. Tomato paste, my dear, not tomato sauce. Leave either one on for at least fifteen minutes before rinsing with warm water and patting dry. I know it sounds weird, but trust me, they both work just like their high-priced counterparts. And the lemons? Cut them in half, place upright on the kitchen counter, then lean over and rest your dry little elbows right on top of them for ten or so minutes before rinsing. Bye-bye old dry skin! Who knew there were such beauty wonders to be found in a grocery store? You may never go to a spa again. ✒

details, details

I'VE GIVEN YOU A WEALTH OF SMALL DETAILS TO FOCUS
attention on, from the way your sheets smell (lavender, I hope)
to the kind of music that runs through your head as you enter
a room (triumphant!). Let me give you one more small thing
to focus on: your shoes. No doubt some of you are already
shoe-obsessed; there are entire television shows devoted to the
passion nowadays. But I'm not talking about the kind of shoes
you choose to wear, or how many pairs line the inside of your
closet. Whatever you wear, I want it to shine! "Unshined shoes
are the end of civilization," said Diana Vreeland. She took her
own maxim to heart so strongly that she even recommended
having the soles shined, lest you "go out to dinner and suddenly lift your foot and the soles aren't impeccable...what
could be more ordinary?" That might be taking
things a bit far (not to mention sounding a

bit slippery). I'm only suggesting that you on occasion indulge in having your shoes shined. Yes, the way men do. The next time you pass a shoeshine booth in an airport, hotel lobby, or side street, take a fifteen-minute break from your ordinary life and hop up there next to the men and settle in. The shoeshine guys will be delighted by your feminine presence. ⌇

only the best

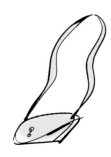

OUR COUNTRY ABOUNDS WITH VARIETY; YOU CAN BUY ANY KIND OF goods and services at an astonishing array of prices. I know I am apt to choose the bargain alternative whenever there is one, but there should be at least one small part of your life in which you will buy only the best. Take a vow that, henceforth, you will settle for only the very best of ____ (and you can fill in this blank any way you desire!). Please don't bankrupt yourself by choosing a big part of your life, such as cars or furniture. Indulge a small part of your life by choosing something such as your underwear, your hair, or your coffee. And then buy only—only and always—the best. Become a connoisseur in whatever area you choose. Know everything about your area, and seek it out everywhere you go. Create trips around it. Have adventures while seeking it out. A friend who had a cancer scare in which it appeared that one of her hands might be amputated, decided after her clean bill of health to "never again buy a cheap purse. Life is just too short to carry a cheap purse." Yes, she will certainly skimp and seek out bargains in other parts of her life, but what she carries in the hands she still has will be top-grade leather from famous designers, by golly. What will it be for you? ☙

mmmmm, what's that smell?

THINK ABOUT THIS: WHAT IF ONE MORNING YOU WOKE UP IN your very own bed, in your very own room, but the air was filled with the incredible aroma of freshly baked bread? Wouldn't that be heavenly? And it seems impossible, unless you live in an apartment over a bakery in Paris. But it's not as impossible as that. All you need is an inexpensive bread machine. Sure, bread machines were pricey when they first came out, but now you can buy them for $50 or so. Simple to operate, it will fill your house with the luxurious scent of baking bread in no time. How do you get to wake up to the smell? You follow the directions for timed baking. Choose a recipe for a breakfast bread, such as raisin walnut, dump in the ingredients, and set the timer the night before according to the instructions. And then, while you sleep and dream, your little bread machine will begin its cycle of kneading, rising, and baking in the middle of the night, so that you can wake up and believe for one fleeting moment that you are in Paris. ❧

the smell of old leather

ONE WAY TO EASILY DESIGN A LIFE THAT MAKES YOU LOOK like a princess at ease in the world, just back from Mombasa, is to decorate with old leather suitcases. You've seen how great they look in the Ralph Lauren ads, or used as displays in department stores, so why not pick up a few yourself and scatter them around your house or apartment? I use them for all kinds of things.

One deep leather hatbox serves as a liqueur bar filled with bottles and special glasses for late-night drinks. Another one holds the family silver (might as well make it easy for a burglar to just pick it up and walk off), and three large leather suitcases are stacked one on top of the other to create an end table. Where do you find them? Probably in your grandparents' garage, or your folks' attic, or a neighborhood garage sale. Trust me, once you develop an eye for it, the world is full of old suitcases. For an old-money luxury touch, try traveling with them! You'll look like an impoverished countess. ❧

apologize, and mean it

AS YOU'VE READ OVER AND OVER IN THE PRECEDING PAGES, luxurious things are often free. They can be thoughts, words, or gestures. And here are two words that qualify: *I'm sorry*. How is apologizing a luxury? Saying "I'm sorry" is a great luxury indeed, if it can solve a problem quickly or smooth over a situation. A dollop of consideration can result in a heap of gratitude.

Apologizing can cement friendships and establish new ones. When you are sure of yourself, and not concerned about having to be "right" all of the time, it is easy to size up a situation, understand that those two simple words will fix it, and offer them up—even though you did nothing wrong! I am certain that the reason I was accepted into the small women's college I attended was that I apologized when it wasn't my fault. I'd been invited to an interview tea with a local alum, who was to pass judgment on me for the acceptance process. She never showed up at the appointed place and time. But I, a young woman of sixteen, realized that I needed to leave a note of apology and suggest that I'd misunderstood the instructions. I hadn't, but I was kind enough to spare an older woman some embarrassment. My acceptance letter arrived the next week. Use this new knowledge to sail through life. ♌

naughty girl!

GO AHEAD, DO SOMETHING NAUGHTY. INDULGE A WHIM. Decide to do something at the last minute. Whether it is plucking a rose from a garden as you are passing and sticking it behind your ear or waltzing out the door without underwear, every so often you should just be impulsive. Do something your own mother would be shocked by! Nothing dangerous or illegal, please, but a little bit of naughty might not be a bad idea. Perhaps buy a book that no one would let you read when you were younger, or wear a color that your mother disapproved of. Me, I smoke the occasional cigar—but don't tell my mother that!

give it up

JUST AS OFFERING THE APOLOGY "I'M SORRY" CAN BE AN indulgence in some situations, so too can saying it to yourself. That's right, I want you to apologize to yourself. Forgive yourself for whatever shortcomings you've had in the past, whatever missteps you've taken, and wherever you feel you've gone wrong. Just forgive yourself and move on into the future, unfettered by guilt and excited about what is to come. We all spend far too many evenings sitting in a funk, rehashing past mistakes and ancient history. Move on. Let yourself off the hook. Decide that you will henceforth lead a different kind of a life—one in which you are certain of your value, your right to go after the things you desire, and your ability to create the life of your dreams. Start right now, don't wait until tomorrow! Why not take out some of that nice stationery you now have and write yourself a kind note of apology. Sign it, seal it up, and send it to yourself to be reread in the moments when you waver. ❧

❧ amongst the flowers

A WELL-TENDED ROSE GARDEN IS A DELIGHT, BUT WHO HAS THE
time or the space? Not I. Thankfully, most cities have a public park
with a lovely rose garden that the taxpayers maintain for you.
Decide that this will be your rose garden, and settle in. Imagine the
calmness that will descend as you stroll slowly down the aisles, sniff-
ing deeply and admiring the beautiful blooms. I'd suggest that you
stay away during the times that public rose gardens are overrun by
brides and grooms and wedding guests, and instead make it a habit
to stop by in the late afternoon and early evening. The sun setting
behind those lovely flowers will create a civilized and luxurious setting. A large group of friends and I moved into a rose garden near
us one summer, some years ago, gathering for weekday potluck
picnics in the early evening. An artist, the fair-haired Cathleen,
showed up once with a lovely and thoughtful touch—she brought
five tiny kittens for us to hold on our laps as we sat there among the
roses. A delicious moment indeed. ❧

steal an afternoon

WHEN WAS THE LAST TIME YOU TOOK YOURSELF OUT TO THE MOVIES? Not with a date, not with your friends, not with your children. Just you and you alone. This is one of my favorite indulgences. Choosing a weepy, romantic movie along the lines of *The Age of Innocence* or *The English Patient*, and sitting alone in the dark sniffling and wiping your nose without worrying if someone might tease you is sheer heaven. Sneak out to see a movie some afternoon by yourself, without telling anyone where you are going. Stop by the snack counter and load up on all of your favorite treats (mine are the malted milk balls). Not only will you get to enjoy a movie that you chose yourself, but you also won't have to share your candy! Settle into those plush seats, shut off your cell phone, forget your worries, and allow yourself to be completely absorbed in another world for just an hour or two. Your life will still be there when you get back, but in the meantime, you can be somewhere else and wonderfully alone with yourself. ❧

dinner at eight

"DRESSING FOR DINNER" IS SUCH AN ELEGANT CUSTOM. Doesn't it evoke grand images in your mind? Dukes and duchesses sweeping down a gilded staircase to sit at a long and elegant table; white-coated footmen standing at attention behind them. Not a scene likely to be found in my home anytime soon, but we can always dream…What I can have at my home, though, is the occasional night when I can convince my husband and children to dress for dinner. Not often, but sometimes. Christmas Eve, New Year's Eve, and once or twice throughout the year, we all gather in our finery and sit down together. It does take a bit of effort to clean the boys' jackets afterwards, but hey, they are getting better every time. You, too, should be able to convince the people in your life to smarten up at dinnertime once or twice a year. It might take bribes and pleading, but hopefully they will play along. As you all sit together, do note how much better behaved we all are when we dress up.

Perhaps that was the reason they did it so many years ago—it made the evening so much more pleasant. So let's all work to bring that back, shall we? ❧

buy original art

DO YOU READ WITH ENVY THOSE MAGAZINE ACCOUNTS OF THE lifestyles of the rich and famous? Such fabulous houses, such beautiful clothes, such handsome children, and all that original art hanging on the walls! Slowly, our houses and our clothes might improve (and I know your children are already handsome), but there is no need to wait to indulge in original art. Start buying now. The idea of art and artists can be so intimidating. Get over it. Artists are people who spend their time hoping you will like their work enough to buy it. They want you; they need you. A wonderful way to buy original art, everything from paintings to sculpture to prints, is to attend charity benefits. For the price of a ticket you'll be able to wander among all kinds of original art that has been donated to the charity in the hopes that people just like you will buy it. In the Pacific Northwest a few months ago, I attended one such event that was jammed with folks eager to buy art at reduced prices. Silent auctions are the best. You just circle around and write in your name and bidding number under the art you like, noting how much you want to spend. And then another art lover comes along and writes her name under yours, upping the bid! So you counterstrike with another, higher bid. It is great fun, kind of competitive, and good for a wonderful story to tell friends about how you came by that particular piece of art.

A WHOLE NEW WORLD

Once you do get in the habit of attending charity art events, think about taking the next step—attending an actual art auction at an auction house, such as Butterfield's or Sotheby's. It is much less formal than the auctions that get big news coverage, such as those selling items that belonged to Jackie Onassis and The Duke and Duchess of Windsor. I bought the travel photos of the Duchess of Windsor at that auction, and it was something of a thrill. But I also get the same thrill every time I open my mailbox and find a catalog from an auction house, or an invitation to come to a reception at an opening night. It really isn't that hard to get on those lists, exclusive as they might sound. And for the twenty minutes you flip through the catalog, you are in a whole different world. You can gain entry to other worlds just as easily by subscribing to unusual journals and newsletters. One of my favorites is *Paris Notes*, a monthly newsletter that is chock-full of tidbits about what is new and exciting in Paris. I hardly ever get a chance to go there, but what a lovely little luxury it is to behave as though I might! For subscription information, go to www.parisnotes.com.

one, two, three; one, two, three

WOULDN'T IT BE SPLENDID TO KNOW HOW TO DANCE ELEGANTLY across the floor, your evening gown shimmering in the lights? Ballroom dancing is all the rage in some places, and chances are there are classes near you. By indulging in ballroom dance lessons, you will not only learn to dance, but you will also trim your figure under that evening gown, work on your posture, and acquire a more graceful way of moving. There is such a romantic air about ballroom dancing—the men seem so courtly and debonair, the women so deliciously dressed. And the audience claps! Once again, you will be doing something that will give you that indescribable thrill of hearing applause for something you are doing. One can never hear enough applause. If you don't know about this world of glamour and romance, rent the movie *Strictly Ballroom*, and see if you get swept up into the idea. I'm guessing you will!

DANCING IN THE DARK

If you can't convince a partner to ballroom dance, I still want you to move and sway to romantic music. It takes two to ballroom dance, but it takes only you to decide to get up and dance by yourself. Let this be the new theme for a life in which you give yourself permission to indulge yourself. Just sway to the music, snap your fingers, and start to dance around the room. Because you aren't afraid. You aren't shy. Your inner princess just got up and walked out onto the dance floor that is your life. Enjoy it for as long as you can. ❧

frankly my dear...

MY GOODNESS, BY THE TIME YOU FINISH THIS BOOK YOUR wardrobe will resemble the costume room on a studio lot from the glamour days of movie-making. Here's one more luxurious item every princess should be able to slip into when the mood strikes—a velvet smoking jacket. Can you picture this? Essentially, it's a basic tuxedo jacket with velvet touches, sometimes a quilted pattern, often a paisley design. Very swank. Wear one and you'll feel like Clark Gable and Carole Lombard rolled into one. Who knows? You might even take up smoking cigars with me. A smoking jacket harkens back to days when men and women separated after dinner, the men to their libraries with cigars and brandy, and the women to their drawing rooms for sherry and gossip. Slip into a velvet smoking jacket and pull on a pair of blue jeans and high heels, or perhaps leggings and mules, and you just might begin to saunter toward the liquor cabinet. As with so many wonderful things in life, look first in a vintage shop or online to pick up one of these goodies. ↔

on the rocks

WE'VE TOUCHED ON MASSAGE AS A DELICIOUS INDULGENCE, AND this new twist on an ancient technique is also well worth trying: hot stone massage. You lie face down on a heated massage table while a talented masseuse leans into your aches and pains with warm oiled rocks, using them to manipulate your pampered

flesh. It's delicious, but it comes with a nearly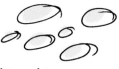
$100 price tag. Is there a way to indulge for
less? Yes, says spa owner and beauty expert
Laura du Priest. She gave me tips on how to achieve this
same effect on your own. I used smooth rocks, heavy massage oil,
thick towels, and a willing partner. Basalt (volcanic) rocks hold
the heat the best, but I bought something called Mexican pebbles
from a local nursery and found they worked just fine. I heated
them (to about 250° F) in a large kettle of water and carefully lifted
them out with a ladle. Be careful and test the heat; never put a rock
on yourself without first checking to see how warm it is! Once
you've determined that the rocks are at a comfortable temperature,
you can try one of two things. Lie down with a warm towel covering your bare skin and have a friend place several of the warm rocks
at various points on your back and shoulders and lie still to absorb
the feeling of warmth, or, have your friend apply oil to your skin
and massage your shoulders and neck with the stones themselves. If
money's no issue, have it done at a spa. ↬

if you can't say something nice....

I'M NO SAINT (IN CASE YOU WERE SOMEHOW MISTAKEN) but I try not to sin too often. And here is a wonderful and saintly good habit to adopt—stay away from gossip. Don't listen to it, don't repeat it, and we can all luxuriate in a bath of kindness toward our fellow women (because you know we hardly ever gossip about men!). Yes, I can't deny that sometimes gossip is naughty good fun. But if you indulge in it often, you just might end up friendless and alone. And if you know your friends indulge in it, you might spend many a sleepless night worrying about what they talk about on the nights you aren't with them....Imagine vowing to indulge in restraint, to be nice, not pass along mean news about acquaintances, and not join in when the talk turns nasty. Wouldn't that be a breath of fresh air in all our lives?

strike a pose

NOT LONG AGO I SAW AN EVOCATIVE AD FOR GUCCI: A WOMAN in a black silk kimono dramatically posed with her arms held up in a languorous position, her wrists heavy with black beaded bracelets that glimmered in the photographer's light. Hmmm...I thought, as I studied the ad. For once, I wasn't looking with envy at her robe, but instead at her bracelets. "I love that look," was my first thought. "I can make those myself," was my second thought, and I was off to the local bead store. Several hours later I emerged, with both wrists filled with the satisfying weight of black beaded bracelets, twenty on each arm. It certainly added a touch of flash to the jeans and sweater I was wearing on an oth-erwise ordinary day. Not only do arms full of beaded bracelets have a satisfying weight to them, but they also move as you do and give you a regal bejeweled feeling that is quite inexpensive. Choose one color, and use several different types of beads so that you end up with bracelets that catch the light. I chose to drape my wrists in black, but you might choose a different color to go with your favorite outfit. As with the velvet smoking jacket, pairing arms full of beaded bracelets with jeans is a dashing look. ⚮

wild things

NOW THAT YOU KNOW ALL ABOUT VINTAGE FUR AND HOW TO BUY it, why not be really bold and decorate with it? I took my husband's mother's old leopard skin coat to the local furrier and for the modest sum of $100, they cut it up and used some of the skin to upholster a footstool. I only wanted that one small fur accent in my house (a little leopard goes a long way, don't you agree?), so I invited a few friends to make their own decorator pillows with the leftovers. If you don't happen to have an old fur hanging in the back of the closet, keep a sharp eye out at garage sales, thrift shops, or online. And you might also convince a few friends to go in and buy one together so that you can each end up with a sumptuous pillow of your own for less. ⚮

comfortably worn

SO MUCH OF WHAT IS ADVERTISED IN MAGAZINES AND SHOWN IN stores is just so...new and shiny. Does everything need to be brand spanking new for us to enjoy it? I don't believe it does. In fact, I purposely seek out things with a bit of patina, such as chairs and dressers and china that were once owned by someone else. As I have politely mentioned once or twice in these pages, a girl could go broke pretty quickly if she succumbs to the desire to live a more luxurious life by rushing out and buying a bunch of dazzling *objets*. Instead, look around for opportunities to add pieces that come with the benefit of age. Wouldn't you rather own something kind of funky and worn that looks as though it might have once lived in a drafty old mansion? Or it may well be that the couch you need to finish your living room has been in your life all along, sitting in the basement of your grandmother's house just waiting for you to dust it off and drape a shawl over the ripped part. The footstool I had re-covered with leopard skin belonged to my grandmother, although I'm sure she would be annoyed that the carved wooden legs are a tiny bit chewed from a long-ago puppy. But that, too, adds charm. Less time spent in department stores and more time spent wandering around garage sales on the weekends will add up to a much more adventurous look. ⚘

material girl

WHILE WANDERING AROUND GARAGE SALES LOOKING FOR wonderful things you can reuse or reupholster, you might also keep an eye open for interesting fabric stores. Shopping for such sumptuous fabrics as silks, velvets (which I know you are now hanging between your rooms instead of using doors), brocades, and jacquards is a heavenly experience. Compared to the cost of many other lovely things, buying fabric by the yard is quite affordable. Indulging your desire to own yards of nubby raw silk in a deep wine color might lead you slowly toward having a skirt made, or covering your own puppy-chewed footstool. Buying fabrics can also be a wonderful hobby to indulge in while traveling. Imagine the beauty of a carefully folded and stacked display of heavy silks on a table that will give you a chance to lead guests through a travelogue of where you have been and what you have seen and the haggling you did in the marketplace in order to buy all of this for just $7. Hemmed pieces of fabric can be draped over tables and couches or even serve as impromptu shawls on drafty evenings. ❧

the well-traveled look

WHEN TRAVELING, I ALWAYS LOOK FOR UNIQUE KEEPSAKES to bring home, small things such as toothpaste. As a result, I've been addicted to the licorice-flavored Elygdium brand of French toothpaste for the past fifteen years, buying it not only in France but also in Singapore and England. And when I wasn't headed to any of those places, I was begging friends headed to France to please bring a few tubes home for me. How lovely it was to have a periodic infusion of the exotic into my ordinary life without even getting on a plane! Make it a habit to give a little money to friends when they travel someplace interesting and request an equally interesting token upon their return. Recently, I authorized a friend headed to India to shop for a long embroidered coat, giving her a range of what I'd happily pay. I also sent along a request to an old boyfriend headed for his ancestral home in Persia (after all, I reminded him, he'd never brought me a darn thing back in the days when we were dating). You could ask your friends to try to find something to add to your collection of exotic fabrics, or to help fill out the wall of leather-bound books you've built. Ask for something small, no one wants to haul back a statue for you. Be prepared to do the same for your friends in return, though. When it's your turn to fly, be sure to offer to find little treasures for them, too. ♨

small, soft, and warm

MY OLDER SISTER ANNE IS A VERY THRIFTY WOMAN, FAR MORE skilled than I in living well within her means. And since we all try to impress our older sisters, here is a little something I thought up as a Christmas gift to gain points. On the verge of tossing out a moth-eaten cashmere turtleneck sweater (before I learned the secret of the rosemary branches which I will soon share with you), I suddenly had a thrifty thought: If I cut off the turtleneck part, could I make it into a cashmere headband? I could, and I did! I was so proud to offer up my little gift to keep Anne's ears warm during Chicago winters that I looked a little closer at the rest of the sweater...what else could I make out of it? Well, a pillow! By cutting up the body of the sweater I was able to rescue enough woven fabric to fashion a small pillow. I even sat in front of the fire one night and stitched it by hand, feeling a sense of communion with the generations of women before me who've bent their heads over a bit of stitching. And I'm hooked. I now look for drastically reduced sweaters on sale racks to make pillows for friends, and I sent a pink-and-purple-striped one off just yesterday to the daughter of a close friend. Who ever would have worn that wacky striped sweater anyway? It was only $12, and making it into a pillow saved it from the bin, I'm quite sure. Look closely at your cashmere or woolen sweaters before tossing them—you might have the makings of some great stuff! ❧

been there, drank that

I AM VERY STERN WHEN IT COMES TO DRINKING, VERY RIGID IN my rules. And my rule is this—drink like a grown-up. I believe it is time for you to get back to basics and drink like a grown-up, too, my dear. Forget about those silly pink drinks you see on television—those women are actresses and their drinks are merely an accent piece. Stand up straight and learn to drink that way. Grown-ups drink gin, and look pretty good doing it. Learn to appreciate the taste of real liquor, the smoky bite of a single malt scotch, the creaminess of small batch bourbon, the icy flavor of imported vodka. Once you abandon the fruit juices and blender and go back to the simple pleasures of a plain martini (gin, please) and scotch on the rocks, you'll have so much more time to spend with your guests and not have to halt conversations while all those frozen drinks whirl. Buy a nice bottle of scotch, a nice bottle of gin, a nice bottle of vodka, and you'll be all set. ❧

silver rings

IF YOU HAVEN'T YET INHERITED THE FAMILY SILVER OR KNOW YOU don't stand a snowball's chance of ever having more than a silver iced teaspoon to your name, don't despair. A relatively inexpensive way to add the soft glow of silver to your dressed-up dinner table is with silver napkin rings. Other people's silver always adds a bit of old money gloss to the look, especially if you have different monograms on each one. Remember the trick with the old linen napkins, how you can make up imaginary ancestors from whom you've inherited? With old monogrammed napkin rings, you can now have twice as many imaginary ancestors for whom to invent stories. My own table is crowded with Gs and Ps and other old family vowels and consonants whose origins have long since faded away. Vowing to search out your own actual monogram could be the basis of a fun treasure hunt to occupy a rainy Saturday afternoon. Find a neighborhood filled with antique stores and visit each one in search of the perfect napkin ring. ❧

the trunk of wonder

WHAT LITTLE GIRL DIDN'T WISH SHE HAD A DRESS-UP trunk filled with yards of costume jewelry and floppy tulle skirts and paper tiaras? I know I wanted one, and had to satisfy my longings by dressing up in my mother's faded purple bridesmaids' dresses over and over again instead of getting to be a gypsy one day and a ballerina the next. But can't we be little girls again now and build ourselves that treasure chest to play in? Jackie Kennedy Onassis had one that she let her grandaughters and their friends rummage through in order to play pirates and treasure hunts up and down the beach. What can you put in yours? Find a battered old trunk at a junk store and start to fill it with whatever strikes your fancy. Once you have a healthy supply of gauzy skirts, feather boas, and old tap shoes, you might share it with your daughters, you might share it with your sons (my chest has a good supply of wooden swords), and you should definitely share it with your grown-up girlfriends during a wild get-together. This time you get to be the gypsy and the ballerina at once! ∾

a gathering of sages

PERHAPS AN ENTIRE TRUNK OF COSTUMES SOUNDS LIKE A BIT much to you. How would you feel about a selection of robes instead? I've encouraged you to begin the habit of changing out of your ordinary clothes and into a voluminous robe at the end of the day, so why not acquire a selection of robes so that you can invite your friends over to join you for an evening of lounging? You could create an entire dinner party around the idea—men could wear Chinese bankers' robes or old silk bathrobes, and you and your friends could stray toward a more velvet approach. Cashmere robes are lovely, but a bit too close fitting and clingy for this kind of an evening. Be sure to warn your friends in advance (because no one enjoys being asked to dress up without warning, and the guests who don't want to do it could skip the evening entirely) and encourage them to dress simply so that the added robes don't make them look bulky. A table full of folks draped in embroidered silks and padded velvet waving their wine glasses in the air and toasting one another will be a rather regal scene, don't you think? ↬

the splendid sky

SOMETIMES NATURE GIVES US THE MOST SUMPTUOUS DISPLAYS of all, if we only remember to look at the sky above us. Several times a year there are meteor showers that fill the sky like sparklers, giving us a rare opportunity to see one shooting star after another. What a sweet way to spend an evening with a lover, lying together on a thick blanket rolled out on the grass, watching the sky explode before your very eyes. Yes, of course you should sometimes share meteor showers with your children, as it is a wonderful way to see science on parade, but do save a night or two for yourself. How do you find out when the showers are likely to appear? The two major showers are Perseid and Leonid, and you can learn more about them online at www.skywatch.com. ↬

teeny, tiny girl

YOU MIGHT HAVE NOTICED THAT I AM A FAN OF MEN'S CLOTHING.
Men look good in it, sure, but I think I look good in it, too.
Men's sweaters, men's shirts, men's robes...I've got a closet full.
I love the simple, clean lines of menswear and all the classic patterns and fabrics, but I like something else about it, too. Have
you ever noticed that when you try on your man's clothes you feel
sort of...small? Doll-like? Teeny, tiny? I'll never be described as
small, but I sure feel that way in my husband's golf sweater hanging down like a tunic. We women go through so much of our
everyday lives feeling a bit too big by most standards, until we slip
into guy's clothing. Ironic, isn't it, that one of the best ways to
feel utterly girly and feminine and slim and petite is to wander
around engulfed in a big sweater. Such a big, luxurious feel, it
makes you feel so tiny and so well cared for. Go
ahead and raid his closet, reaching deep into the

back for the stuff he doesn't wear anymore, anyway. What, the striped sweater his dotty aunt sent for Christmas six years ago or the oversized Oxford cloth with the button-down collar he hasn't worn since casual Friday has disappeared for good? Then march into the men's department and start choosing menswear in the colors and styles you really want for yourself! ♠

your mona lisa smile

DREAM WITH ME HERE...CENTURIES FROM NOW, AS ART PATRONS peer carefully at the portrait on display in a museum and wonder what was that woman thinking about as she gazed so calmly at the painter, imagine that the delicately rendered woman they gaze upon is...you. Yes, you. Well, why not? Why shouldn't a princess like you be portrayed by artists? You are a lovely creature, and you deserve it. Posing for a portrait needn't be so far-fetched; it could happen to you very easily. Chances are you know someone who paints. Ask if you can pose for him or her. Do you live near a college? Art classes frequently need live models, and you don't always have to take your clothes off. As someone who has taken her clothes off for artists, though, I can assure you that it isn't as racy as it sounds. Artists are much more concerned with getting the lines of your body just right than trying to seduce you. Not long ago, a local artist for whom I posed years ago had an exhibit at a nearby museum and I went straightaway to his show, desperately hoping that my nude portrait wouldn't be hanging there on the wall for all to see, and then was a bit disappointed to learn that it wasn't. ৵

honestly luxurious

WE HOLD SO MUCH INSIDE OF US, DON'T WE? WE TRY TO KEEP so many of our real and honest feelings and impressions bottled up inside of us, either because we want to keep the peace at home or because we fear the damage we might do if we unleashed an honest remark. How much longer can we hold this inside? Well, don't. Don't hold your honest thoughts and feelings alone inside of you; write them down in a journal. Use a personal journal as the one place you can indulge in everything you are too polite to share with those around you. Be honest and open on the page; you might even try your hand at secret poetry. Once you find your honest voice in your writing, it might also help you find ways to express yourself more openly with those around you. As with your dream journal, find the most attractive blank journal you can and treat yourself to a special pen that you reserve for this ritual. Keep your journal in a special place and make certain that everyone else in your house understands that it is off-limits, that these are your own private thoughts and not meant to be shared. ❧

a bag of buried treasure

ONCE AGAIN, I'D LIKE TO INVOKE THAT LITTLE GIRL YOU ONCE were, the one who really did hope she was a lost princess whose real family would be showing up any time now to claim her...did you ever dream about a bag of treasure? A velvet bag filled to over-flowing with gold coins, maybe a few diamonds thrown in for good measure? I can't help you with the diamonds, but I can tell you how to bring that bag of treasure to life now! Paper money is all very well and good, but there is something about coins that makes money feel so much more real. Sacajawea and Susan B. Anthony were both honored with dollar coins that you can still find in circulation. I've recently begun to collect them, even to sometimes ask for my change in dollar coins so that I can add to my hefty stash. It is such a thrilling feeling to have a bag of heavy coins. Not much in actual dollars, just $30 or so for now, but my plan is to gradually grow my sack of coins for the next few years until someday—surprise!—I will present it to someone who needs it. It really is a velvet treasure bag I'm using, one with a golden cord to tie it closed. And I look forward to the day when I pull my bag from its hiding place to share my treasure with another princess. ⟨⟩

alter ego

I'VE ALREADY URGED YOU TO CHOOSE ANOTHER, MORE adventurous name for yourself at this stage of your life. To choose a new moniker—such as the name I choose at age 40, Gin—that better captures who you think you are. But not everyone is ready for that drastic step, so why not take a smaller step. Why not develop an online name that symbolizes your essence? My e-mail address is onedry-martini@hotmail.com. Perhaps you'd like to recast yourself in a different role too. Instead of being someonesmom@boringe-mailaddress.com, you could be salsalover, or speedracer or parisbound. Or maybe you lean more towardredwine, rosepetal, or princessanne. How is this an indulgence, you ask? Because it gives you a chance to indulge (and reveal) your own feelings about yourself and your interests, instead of trapping you in the vision your parents had of who you would be so long ago. Naming yourself to the world can be a wonderful way to fly your own flag, to announce your talents and your strengths. Don't be shy now—create your own world. ❧

never enough, never enough

ALLOW ME TO QUOTE EXTENSIVELY FROM HENRY JAMES'
delightful book *The Europeans*, which every princess of good breed-
ing should read. You will then see immediately that many
princess home decorating policies have their roots in his views:
" *'Il faudra,'* said Augustine, *'lui faire un peu de toilette.'* And she began
to hang up *portieres* in the doorways; to place wax candles…in
unexpected situations; to dispose of anomalous draperies over
the arms of sofas and the backs of chairs. The Baroness had
brought with her to the New World a copious provision of the
element of costume; and the two Miss Wentworths [Charlotte
and Gertrude], when they went to see her, were somewhat bewil-
dered by the obtrusive distribution of her wardrobe. There were
India shawls suspended, curtain-wise, in the parlour door, and
curious fabrics…tumbled about in sitting places…'I have been
making myself a little comfortable,' said the Baroness, much to

the confusion of Charlotte, who had been on the point of proposing to come and help her put her very superfluous draperies away. But what Charlotte mistook for an almost culpably delayed subsidence Gertrude very presently perceived to be the most ingenious, the most interesting, the most romantic intention. 'What is life, indeed, without curtains?' she secretly asked herself; and she appeared to herself to have been leading hitherto an existence singularly garish and totally devoid of festoons." So festoon away, my dear, festoon away. ❧

an evening of art play

SOME MONTHS AGO, AN ARTIST FRIEND INVITED A LARGE GROUP OF women to her house for what we thought was an ordinary get-together of wine and cheese. It was far from ordinary, though, as we learned the minute she plopped a big block of wet clay in the middle of the table and urged us to dive in. Dive in we did, and spent many happy hours sculpting our own self-portraits. Most of us had no idea what we were doing artistically, but it didn't seem to matter. We just loved the play involved. To indulge one's creative side is a luxury indeed, particularly when you know you won't be graded on it! How can you give yourself the permission to create? Buy clay and begin to sculpt whatever you'd like, even if the best you can do at first is to make clay worms and curl them up into bowls. The very act of getting your hands dirty with art will send you straight back to your messy and unrestrained childhood; I'm sure that you will soon be building with imagination and creativity. If clay sounds too yucky, pick up a box of paints and see what you can do. The point is to allow yourself to do whatever comes out without judging it. Let your imagination soar and see where it can take you! ⋆

banish moths with rosemary

NOW THAT YOU HAVE A CLOSET PACKED WITH CASHMERE, HOW DO you keep it princess-perfect? Few things are as heart-stopping as the sight of a tiny hole in your favorite sweater. Just because you now know how to turn an old cashmere sweater into a snug headband and a decorative pillow doesn't mean you want your entire wardrobe to end up that way! Mothballs are smelly, and cedar is expensive. What's a girl to do? Simple. Just go out to the garden and snip some rosemary. I've battled those hungry moths myself and was delighted to learn that fresh rosemary wards off the little guys. Cut yourself a few stalks (or pick them up in the herb section of the grocery store if you don't have rosemary growing) and place them in and around your sweaters. You might also cut a nice bunch and wrap the ends in twine and hang it upside down in your closet. Cutting fresh rosemary and replacing it every few weeks is a nice little ritual that gets you out into your garden, and the real bonus is that your closet smells like an Italian bakery all the time. Ahhhh, fresh focaccia! What could be better? ⟊

morning, or afternoon of the faun

EVERY MORNING IT HAPPENS. HEART RACING, YOU JOLT AWAKE to the loud sound of a buzzer or a blast of music. Not a very peaceful and relaxing way to start your day, is it? Why not find a way to slowly and gently wake up. Hiring a handsome tuxedo-clad man to do the job every morning would be lovely, but in the absence of that, get yourself a small CD player with a gradual alarm. The kind that starts off kind of low and quiet and then gradually increases to the point where your subconscious mind is finally (but gently) aware of it. Bose makes this exact type of alarm and I highly recommend it. You've noticed before that my philosophy on spending money focuses on finding some small luxury—such as a small, high-end radio/CD—and putting it someplac where you can really enjoy it. Instead of silly shock jock talk on a rude radio station, imagine instead that you are slowly waking to the strains of Debussy's "Afternoon of the Faun," or "La Mer," or some other lovely piece that can nudge you awake every morning. Delicious...particularly if you've learned to program a bread machine! ⚬⚭

a trip around the world

ONCE I TRAVELED WITH A LOVER TO PARIS, REJOICING IN THE sights and sounds of that enchanted city. He was in Paris for three weeks, but the fact is I never really left home. How'd that work? The entire time he was walking the streets of Paris I was absorbed in a Balzac novel that led me down those same streets. So when he returned, I felt like I'd been there with him the entire time. Why not try this yourself, traveling to whichever city your heart most yearns to see. Venice? Sit down and read Marlena de Blasi's *A Thousand Days in Venice* with wineglass in hand, and you will emerge from the pages believing you have lived alongside her. Seek out novels set in Bangkok, Rome, Stockholm, London, or whatever your dream destination may be. Devote an entire year to "traveling abroad" by constructing a journey on the page that moves you from country to country. You might find yourself branching out into biographies, or histories, or travelogues—anything that increases your knowledge and enhances the feeling that you've *been* somewhere when you set that book down on your nightstand. ❧

a topping for all occasions

I PLAN TO FURTHER EXPAND YOUR LUXURIOUS COOKING HABITS by sharing my own recipe for an incredible dessert sauce, one that will delight and amaze your family or your guests. Once you've mastered this simple recipe you'll be able to whip it up at a moment's notice and add a gloss of goodness to the most ordinary ice cream, cookies, or pies. Since it has four ingredients and each one pretty much calls for $1/4$ cup, I've always referred to this as "Four by Four Sauce," but that really doesn't sound posh enough for the purposes of this book. So henceforth, it shall be known as "A Quatre Sauce." That's French for "foursome," in case you weren't paying attention in class.

All you need are four things—unsalted butter, white sugar, brown sugar, and cream. In a pinch I've used milk, but nothing beats cream. And then you need $1/4$ cup of each of those ingredients (see how easy it will be to remember this when you are visiting a friend's house and suddenly feel the urge to impress?). In a teflon saucepan melt the butter over medium heat, then add the two kinds of sugar. Stir until they are well melted and mixed. Pour in the cream and mix well. Here is the slightly scary part—bring the sauce to a boil and leave it alone for one to two minutes; resist the urge to stir. Should you wish to change the *quatre* to a *cinq*, feel free to add a tablespoon of almost any type of liquor. Bourbon is delightful, as is cognac. ⟨♠⟩

drift off to sleep

WHILE WE ARE ON THE TOPIC OF HIGH-CALORIE INDULGENCES, I'd like to share my favorite sleep-inducing beverage. Ah, you're guessing it is a slug of bourbon, but you'd be wrong! No, it is an innocent carryover from childhood—a glass of warm malted milk. Science is on my side with this one; calcium really does have sleep-inducing abilities. My brand of choice is Horlick's, which I was introduced to decades ago when an English cousin tucked me into bed with a glass after a long flight to the British

Isles. It was heaven. And so began my devotion to a mug of Horlick's and warm milk at night. However was I to keep a supply on hand, though? I packed the sides of my suitcase with glass jars and prayed they wouldn't burst during the journey. Sadness set in when I noticed my supply dwindling, because I had neither the means nor the time to plan another trip to England. And then I looked a little more closely at one of those jars I'd lovingly brought back to the States. Made in Ohio. Oh. So you shouldn't have any problem finding it on the shelves of a grocery store. Stir it into warm milk just as you would hot chocolate, carry that mug to bed and climb in. ✿

sashay by the pool

LOOKING FOR A FAST WAY TO FEEL LIKE A MILLION DOLLARS? There is one way to instantly feel sexy, slim, and mysterious. Simply don your swimsuit, slip on high heels, and tie a sarong around your waist. It doesn't matter what your body shape is or what size your bathing suit is, you will feel like a movie star. That

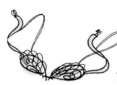 sarong will make you feel amazing...your bottom and the tops of your thighs are covered (so there's one less thing to worry about), but there is just something about the jaunty angle at which it is tied that makes you feel wonderful. For maximum glamour, stretch out on a lounge chair by the pool for the day. Rub on expensive suntan lotion (really, it just smells better than the cheap stuff, but we are all about creating atmosphere here, so please do indulge and spend the extra $3), and come equipped with a wide-brimmed hat and enough glossy magazines to last for hours. I'm not suggesting that you actually swim, but if you do, make sure it is a slow breaststroke and wear your sunglasses and hat the whole time. ⚘

oh, you are soooo manly

ON A FIRST DATE LONG AGO, I ASKED MY NEW FRIEND WHAT THAT heavenly smell was. Hermés' Caliche, he told me. There in the dark movie theater my eyebrows raised in sheer surprise as I thought to myself, "Hey, but that's perfume!" I didn't go out with him again (he was an unemployed poet), but it did open up a whole new world of scent to me. The very next day I marched into a department store and bought myself a bottle of Eau Sauvage, a sexy lemony men's fragrance. Most perfumes had always been a touch too flowery for me anyway, and once I realized Nick was wearing perfume without anyone questioning his masculinity, I figured no one would dare assume that I was wearing a man's scent. And I was right; no one ever sniffed and said, "Ew! Are you wearing men's cologne?!" From the lemony scent of Eau Sauvage I moved on to the piney smell of Aqua di Selva and from there to what I still wear today—Ralph Lauren's Safari for Men. Is it any cheaper? Quite a bit, in fact, and a bottle of men's cologne seems to last much longer than those teeny girl's perfume bottles. ∞

the bathing tradition

MY SISTER ANNE IN CHICAGO INTRODUCED ME TO THIS DELICIOUS indulgence—an evening at the Japanese Baths. Many religions have cleansing rituals for women, and many countries such as Russia and Turkey have traditions where public baths are gathering places for both sexes to while away the afternoon or evening. This is not, then, the place to take a date. A Japanese bathhouse is the place to plan an evening with your girlfriends or to spend time with yourself. Naked. In a room full of strangers. Moving back and forth between the hot pool and the cooler pool, and then finishing up with a shower. This is not a pursuit for shy girls, but for women who feel comfortable with their bodies. Even if you feel awkward about your size, you still might give this a try; the room will be filled with women's bodies of all sizes. In a Japanese bath it is part of the ritual to soap up and rinse off *first*, before getting into the tub. You'll enjoy the mindless leisure of just sitting and soaking away your cares, all the while stimulating your circulation and relaxing those aches and pains. Some bathhouses even have masseuses on staff to add to the experience. This costs extra, though. Without the massage a typical evening at a Japanese bathhouse is around $30 and well worth it. ❧

escape into a book

I FIRMLY BELIEVE THAT THE MOST LUXURIOUS WAY TO SPEND an afternoon or evening is planted in a comfy chair, lost in a book. Any book. Novels, biographies, travel accounts, history, cookbooks, whatever strikes your fancy, just read. Read often, read always, read everywhere. Reading can do so many luxurious things for you—take you far away from your daily struggles, give you a glimpse into other worlds, teach you things you might otherwise never learn. Among my useless pieces of knowledge is that before Jakarta, Indonesia, was called Jakarta, it was called Batavia. Might that come in handy someday? One never knows, does one? I once won a pot of money on a game show because I knew that "Ghiradelli" was the answer to the question "Name a 150 year old chocolate company." Reading widely gives you confidence in the world and the firm sense that you are not alone, no matter how suddenly unbearable your life might seem. Don't forget what Voltaire (you might try reading him, too) said: *"Let us read and let us dance—two amusements that will never do any harm to the world."* ❧

assemble your court

NOW THAT YOU'VE TAKEN UP WEARING A ROBE AND MOVING regally from room to room, why not take this princess life one step further by creating your very own court? Hey, it worked for the Sun King; you've seen how lovely it all looked at Versaille. Sadly, you won't have much luck pressing your friends and family into acting as handmaidens or ladies-in-waiting, but you will get them to fall into line once you start awarding them titles. Take a page from the imaginative folks at the Society for Creative Anachronism and anoint everyone around you. Christmas Eve at my house finds my family assembled around a beautifully laid table, dressed in our Renaissance finery. My sons, momentarily answering to the names Lord Julian and Sir Pips, wear velvet tunics and wooden swords. I confess that the gentleman of the house won't play along with this fantasy and not everyone in your life will, either. But some of your friends might want to be royals for the night. Why not throw a soiree and invent names and titles for everyone? Write out the fancy names and the descriptions of their new identities and hand them out when your guests arrive. It will make the beginnings of a grand and memorable evening! ⚘

a day by the sea

OUR MEMORIES OF TRAVEL ARE AMONG THE MOST PRECIOUS. STORE up your impressions of beloved destinations so that you can close your eyes at will and conjure up a lazy scene at a favorite café in a far-flung town at a moment when all else in your life seems to be going wrong. And don't just bring your memories home, bend down and pick up a few seashells, some smooth stones, or a tiny pinecone that you can display in a corner of your home to remind yourself in between visits. In my guest bathroom, I have a blue glass jar filled to the brim with seashells from long ago Mexican beaches. On the top of a chest of drawers sits a collection of petrified seashells that were given to us as a gift on our honeymoon in Thailand ("may your marriage last as long as these million-year-old shells," the driver said, as he handed them to us, which even in the throes of a romantic honeymoon sounded like a bit much to me). You might already have a stash of shells somewhere in your house from a trip. Take them out and place them in a lovely dish to give yourself a visual vacation every time you notice them. Stones and rocks are just as pretty as shells. One friend collects beach glass and shows it off in jars placed near a window to catch the light. Whatever you collect from your trips, give it pride of place. Keep the feeling of adventure going. ⚓

only the best for you

FUZZY SLIPPERS ARE A MUST FOR A PAMPERED PRINCESS. YOUR delicate feet must be protected from the elements at all times, encased in a froth of faux fur or puffy feathers. For in-house use, I'll look the other way while you pass on the high heels, as there are many times in life when a girl needs to keep her feet firmly on the ground, and first thing in the morning is certainly one of them. Slippers do seem so mundane, though. Is there a way to move them farther down luxury lane? *Bien sur*, as the French say. But of course. Not long ago, I bought myself some purple felt spa booties that come with a liner of lavender seeds. Pop them into the microwave for a minute or so, slip them onto your already lotioned feet, and ah...heaven. A bit crunchy to walk in, but the point here is not to walk so much as to recline regally, your pampered feet raised in the air and propped on a lovely footstool. Sounds so decadent, and well worth it if you can track them down. Is there a way to feel this way without the spa booties? Sure. Just choose your thickest, most luxurious cotton socks, sprinkle them with a few drops of water to moisten, and pop them into the microwave. Slather lotion on your feet while they are warming up, then pull the toasty socks on right away. Alas, the warmth doesn't last long, but it feels delicious. If you can't find the spa booties in a store near you, try www.redenvelope.com. ❧

would you care for a taste?

WE WORK SO HARD TO ENTERTAIN OURSELVES SOMETIMES, WHY not relax and let someone else do the work for you? Why not take advantage of all those hardworking folks with little wine shops who devote their Friday evenings or late Saturday afternoons to holding tastings for the public? I'm not suggesting that you take advantage of them financially; I do think you should buy their wares. But I am suggesting that you sit down and relax and let someone else pour you a taste of wine, then talk to you about where it came from and how it was made. Take advantage of their wish to cultivate you as a customer, to teach you what they know, to spark in you a desire to learn more about the world of wine, to come back to their little shop again and again. It can be a lively way to pass the time, meeting new people and talking about new things. Wine folks are fascinating. They know about food, geography, climate, languages, and history. Shouldn't you?

Once you attend a tasting event or two, make sure you get added to the mailing list so that you will be invited to smaller, less public events. ❧

a slogan of one's own

"YOU CAN NEVER BE TOO RICH OR TOO THIN." YOU RECOGNIZE that saying, don't you? Ah, but do you know who said it? It has long been attributed to one of my own lux idols, the Duchess of Windsor. She worked very hard at both thinness and richness. Amusing as that slogan is, I would never adopt it as my own. Clearly my own devotion to chocolate and cream will stop me far short of thinness. No, my own slogan is "Red Wine, Black Dresses," which neatly sums up my approach to life. Why don't you create a slogan that embraces your beliefs? Don't let the folks at Nike ("Just do it!") have all the fun. Try not to stray into the mom or wife territory; choose a phrase that celebrates you for being you, rather than you in relationship to others. Something that highlights your devotion to a hobby, such as, "So many books, so little time." Or for a beach lover, perhaps something like, "To the sea!" Once you've developed a slogan, make sure you use it! Print it on your business card, embroider it on your sheets, needlepoint it on your pillows. Don't put it on your license plate, though; that's a bit too lowbrow for a princess. ⚓

why wait? start with the pie!

YES, I DO LIKE A SWEET OR TWO. I AM TERRIBLY RESTRAINED, though, compared to my friend Sherry. You have a Sherry in your life, too, I suspect. Someone who prefers to indulge in chocolate and ice cream and seldom gets around to her vegetables (but looks like a supermodel nevertheless). Early on I suggested that you shake things up a bit by starting with a glass of champagne before dinner instead of after. Why not shake things up further by having dessert first? Who said you always have to wait for dessert until the end, anyway? Make your own rules, be bold. On Sherry's 30th birthday, she ordered two desserts and had them brought when the rest of us had our soups and salads. Who do you think enjoyed the evening more? Those of us who dutifully had a bit of greens and veg before our sweet, or the woman who plunged right in? You might also try the approach of Clare Boothe Luce, a glittering personality from the twenties who started out as a magazine editor (*Vanity Fair*), became a playwright (*The Women*) and ended up as Ambassador to Italy in the seventies, would often lunch on plain lettuce leaves and then dig into a healthy slice of apple pie. 🍎

to sleep, perchance to dream...

I'D SEEN THE ADS FOR YEARS, THERE IN THE IN-FLIGHT CATALOG next to the airline magazine. It sounded so compelling to someone stuck in a tiny coach seat...a silk dream sack. A tiny silk sleeping bag, really, meant to be slipped in between your own dull sheets so that your delicate skin is swathed at all times in the luxury and warmth of whisper-thin spun silk. Ah...it sounded heavenly. But a bit much, really. Did I really need this in my life? One afternoon on a particularly uncomfortable flight to Chicago, I finally broke down and called. The very thought that a midnight blue DreamSack was now on its way to me kept me going for the rest of the ghastly plane flight. Days later a package arrived. Would it really be all that I'd dreamed of those past few years? It was. If you are reading this book while sitting on a plane, my heart goes out to you, dear. Reach into the seat pocket in front of you and flip through that shopping catalog until you find the ad for DreamSack, and focus on that image of luxury until your plane lands. If you aren't on a plane, check out the Web site at www.comfortchannel.com, or call 1-800-303-7574. It is far less than the cost of high-cotton sheets, and you might find you don't even need expensive sheets once you have a DreamSack. Slip in and dream away. ᴧ

act as if!

TAKING A PAGE OUT OF THE PLAYBOOK OF MANY A MOTIVATIONAL speaker, I am here to tell you that you should act *as if* your life is exactly the way you want it to be. Your own thoughts can make a tremendous difference in your present happiness, so why not indulge in *as if* thoughts and behaviors? Not happy with your present size and working to slim it down? Act *as if* you are already thin, think *as if* you are already at your target weight, and you will be halfway there. Walk into a crowded room *as if* you were the honored guest, and you soon will be. When it comes to a regal approach to life, act *as if* you are indeed a princess, and you will be one! Remember that being a princess in the "wear more cashmere" sense is not about ordering people around or demanding to be treated in a special way. It is about you treating yourself in a special way. Treating yourself *as if* you were born to the manor will at the very least get you in the same neighborhood as one. ⚘

from the library of...

NOW THAT YOU ARE TRAVELING THE WORLD THROUGH BOOKS, please do clear out space on your shelves and establish a beautiful library of your own. Choose a theme to your books, deciding only to collect only books about Paris, for instance, or opera singers, or the Civil War, or whatever quirky personal interests you have. My own library includes an enormous collection of literature about traveling to China in the twenties and thirties (research for a very naughty novel I plan to write someday) and a good-sized collection of books about Chanel. For years, writer Harriet Rubin collected tales of strong women leaders throughout history and ultimately turned them into a book called *The Princessa*. Of course, your shelf will be packed with the books you pick up and read throughout the course of a year, but make it a point to give your collection pride of place. Perhaps you can find bookends to mark off the space, bookends that somehow symbolize what your collection is all about. You can also take your new family crest, or your newly created slogan, and design a bookplate for yourself to paste inside each book in your library. You'll come to relish this new hobby of seeking out books for your collection. It will take to you far-flung places, in and out of incredible used bookshops, and online to find tidbits of information from other collectors. ⚓

the jardin coiffure

I ONCE HAD MY EYE ON A HANDSOME ARTIST, A PAINTER WHO WAS much sought after by the women in my artsy crowd. How could I catch his eye when there were always so many other women around? I took to appearing at parties wearing one white gardenia pinned in my hair. Every time I walked past, he would catch a small whiff of my flower and turn to watch. It took a whole summer of picking flowers from my front yard, but my efforts finally paid off. Even if you aren't trying to attract one particular man, you will feel like a star with a flower tucked in your hair. Orchids and gardenias both work nicely, and camellias are also a good choice. Baby's breath is best left to young high school girls on their way to the prom, and roses don't last that well. Look first in your own garden to see what you can experiment with before asking a friendly florist for recommendations. Try it, and you will immediately feel sensual and exotic. And take it from me, with a flower in your hair, men will follow you wherever you care to lead them. ⋗

and what would you like to do today?

TRAVEL IS WONDERFUL; IT PRESENTS AN ENDLESS CHANCE TO GO new places, see new things, and meet new people. Alas, when we travel with others, though, most of the time we are going to the places they want to go, seeing the things they want to see, and meeting the people *they* want to meet. Sigh. I speak from experience; take it from a woman who has ridden on steam trains in most of the lower forty-eight states. And no, stream trains are not my hobby. I'd much prefer to spend the day in a quiet museum or seeking out a performance of a local string quartet. Which is exactly what I do when I travel by myself, and why I highly recommend that you give yourself the opportunity to travel alone sometime. When traveling alone, you don't have to indulge the needs and desires of others, just yourself. Doesn't that sound like heaven? You can check out that antique store without glancing down at your watch, worried that there is someone outside drumming his fingers on the steering wheel. You won't have to get up early to meet someone else's schedule, you won't have to hide the fact that you're dying to try a piece of that famed strawberry-rhubarb pie with double scoops of French vanilla ice cream, and you won't have to sit through a narrated film on famous Civil War battles. Get out the maps, clear some time on your calendar, and announce to the world that you are leaving *by yourself* for a while! ⏺

brows of distinction

WOMEN OF STYLE HAVE SUCH MEMORABLE FACES, OR MAYBE just their eyes are memorable. Or maybe, just maybe, it is their eyebrows that we remember. When deciding just how to divvy up my pampering dollars, I always vote for putting it into a big bang. A facial is a lovely idea, but who other than you will know you've had one? And a few days later will you be able to tell the difference? Not likely. But your brows, now there is a place you can spend a small bit of money and achieve a lasting and noticeable effect! My own brows are pale and skimpy things, but for $25 I can have beautifully dark brown brows that frame my eyes, arched and waxed to perfection and lasting for weeks. This is a movie star treatment, as you lie back on a massage table and trust the shaping and coloring of your eyebrows to a stranger with a degree from a beauty school...Don't despair one minute longer over your scruffy brows. Once you are accustomed to having strangers poke around your delicate eye area, you might also consider another glamour touch—false eyelashes. Celebs like Sarah Jessica Parker, Debra Messing, and Natalie Portman weren't born with longer, darker eyelashes than you and me—they paid extra to have them applied by a makeup artist. Why not give it a try yourself? ❧

through the museum slowly

MUSEUMS ARE A LOVELY PLACE TO SPEND A LAZY AFTERNOON wandering from room to room. What if instead, though, you decided to devote an entire year to getting to know your local museum, room by room? Imagine this: Spend an hour or two every few weeks in a different room in your local art museum, getting to know the individual paintings and their moods. Sit and soak up the beauty at your own pace, instead of moving from the Impressionist room to the Old Masters hall, then walking past the place where they keep the armor on your way to see a Warhol litho or a Lucien Freud portrait. Is that really the way to learn? No. I sat once for an hour in front of an enormous tapestry at the Metropolitan Museum in New York. The tiny information card said it had been woven by nuns in the sixteenth century, and so I sat there solemnly considering the lives of the women whose hands had produced this lasting work of beauty. Who were they? What had they been thinking about as they bent over the loom? Did they talk to each other, or was the work all done in silence? And then I let my mind wander slowly to consider the place where the finished tapestry had originally hung. A castle, I imagined, kind of a big one at that. It was so relaxing to sit and contemplate just one piece of art, rather than try to absorb all of what was there around me. Try this in your favorite museum. Give yourself permission to look at only one piece of art and get to know it. Think about it. Learn what attracts you to it. Go home and research the artist. And then go back the next week and choose a new object or room to study. ◆

a simple indulgence

SHALL I SHARE MY SECRET RECIPE FOR A PERFECT DESSERT? A little luxury for those nights when you might crave chocolate but be a bit too tired to wade through the recipe for homemade chocolate pudding I keep urging on you? Don't despair, help is nearby. Here is a simple indulgence—a glass of red wine and a handful of M&Ms. See how very simple it is? A life of luxury need not be complicated, and it need not be expensive. It need only be delicious! On the spur of the moment, I've invited friends over to join me on the couch at night after the kids are in bed for M&Ms and a glass of wine. It also seems to be a simple dessert that men enjoy (they aren't always so interested in the recipes we work so hard to master, although the chocolate pudding is a man thing, too). One friend came already dressed in her flannel pajamas, unable to resist the idea of a simple chocolate treat. Must I point out that you shouldn't indulge in the M&Ms too often, lest your cashmere grows a tiny bit tight? All luxury is best taken in small doses. ᏈᎲ

dreaming is free

REMEMBER THAT DECORATED DREAM JOURNAL I INSISTED YOU start? The fancy gold-encrusted one in which you could record your dreams and remind yourself that your brain was capable of great flights of creativity? Well, now that you are in the habit of recording your dreams, don't just stop with your unfettered night-time dreams. Continue the practice with your eyes wide open, too. Dream. Indulge your imagination. Don't be afraid to let your mind wander and imagine a different way of life. Indulge not just your imagination but also your hopes and dreams for a different kind of life. Don't ever believe that the life you have now is the only one you will ever know, particularly if you are unhappy with it. No one can stop you from dreaming and planning a different kind of life, and giving yourself the freedom to write it down will give you the courage to take action. Dreaming is free. ⚘

your future file

HERE IS A WAY TO TAKE YOUR WAKING DREAMS ONE STEP further—start building files for them. Once you write down the hopes and dreams you have for your life, start to collect information and make a plan that will actually take you there. I'm not saying you have to share it with anyone. This is your secret stuff, not to be shared unless you feel like it. Wish you could spend a year in Paris? Mark a fresh PARIS file and start to collect brochures for study abroad programs, or apartment rental agencies, or a review of Adam Gopnick's delightful book *Paris to the Moon* (he got to spend much more than a year there!). Or is your secret dream to build a kiln and fire your own pots? Start that file of kiln designs! Me, I have a secret plan to someday have a ranch called "Taschengeld," which I will design and then hand build everything from the stone fences to the guest houses. Yes, I have files with outdoor fireplace designs, land prices, and techniques for building small houses. It might happen, it might not, but in the meantime I will have had tremendous enjoyment thinking about the possibility and gathering information to make it real. Indulge your dreams, my dear, because no one else will indulge them for you. ⁂

hot chocolate for the body

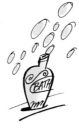

IS THERE A WAY TO ENJOY CHOCOLATE WITHOUT HAVING TO WORRY about our waistlines for once? In fact, there is! Why not immerse yourself in one giant cup of hot chocolate? Instead of pouring yourself a mug, you can mix up a sinfully scented bath that will let you relax amidst the aroma of chocolate. Here is the recipe: You'll need 2 tablespoons of an inexpensive brand of unsweetened cocoa powder (because you don't want to be dumping the pricey stuff into your bath, for heaven sakes!), 1/2 cup of dry milk powder, and 1/2 cup of unscented bubble bath. Toss the ingredients under the tap of a hot running bath and mix it with your hands to make sure there aren't any clumps. Now, what about marshmallows? I recommend saving that until the end, when you are wrapped in a towel and relaxing afterward, and *then* you can enjoy a little sweet to eat! ∿

the musical back rub

A MUSICAL BACKRUB? YES, IT IS A PHRASE COINED BY PETER (you never know when men will suddenly spout something unexpectedly romantic and sweet—that's part of their charm) to describe the act of lying quietly in the dark listening to a piece of incredible music. The musical backrubs in our house are almost always either a Rachmaninoff piano concerto (a more luxurious sound you will never find!) or the soundtrack to the French film *Chocolat*. Your own favorite music will no doubt spring to mind when you imagine your own musical backrub. Make sure it is a piece with enough depth to keep you interested for a solid twenty or thirty minutes. This is an actual backrub, mind you, one that occurs deep within as you lie back and focus just on the music. Don't focus on your day, on your

family, on your unpaid bills. Clear your mind completely. Relax
in the dark, letting the music pour over you. ♪

the red carpet club

IT IS A MAINSTAY OF EVERY AWARDS SHOW—THE WALK DOWN THE
red carpet into the theater. Every actress, television celebrity, or
fading beauty indulges in that slow stroll in front of the cameras,
smiling from side to side and waving grandly at their fans lined
up alongside. What a moment that must be! Is there a way for
you, a way for us, to capture a little bit of the glory of that
moment in our humdrum lives? Yes. Create your own red carpet moment just before you enter a room. You've read here
about the importance of posture, about the luxury of moving
slowly, about how holding your head high and believing in yourself can make all the difference. So why not put all of those things
together and enjoy an imaginary moment before the photographers and the adoring fans? The next time you are about
to enter a crowded meeting room, stop and pause for a

moment. Straighten your spine. Throw back your shoulders. Lift your head. Fasten a small, shy smile on your lips. And then walk straight through that door as if you knew that applause and cheers awaited you on the other side. Make your entrance. Leave your mark. And enter a room as though you own the darn thing. ❧

the four basic food groups

I WILL NOW END MY LESSON ON THE FOUR LUXURY FOOD GROUPS— to the dessert sauce, lobster bisque, and chocolate pudding recipes you now have I am adding a cheese soufflé. The cashmere foods, shall we say. Once you've mastered these few delicious treats, you will be able to casually delight your friends or your loved ones, whipping up a little something to reward their taste-buds at the end of a long day. Soufflés sound so difficult, and many of them are. This one, however, is simple and satisfying, and you will serve it often with a tossed green salad and a bottle of tremendous white wine.

Simple Cheese Soufflé

4 tablespoons butter plus extra for buttering dish
1/4 cup flour
1 1/2 cups whole milk
1 1/2 cups Cheddar cheese
1 tablespoon sweet mustard
salt and pepper to taste
6 eggs, separated

Preheat your oven to 400° F and generously butter an 8" by 12" glass baking dish. In a saucepan on the stovetop, melt the 4 tablespoons of butter over moderate heat on the stove, then add the flour. Whisk it while continuing to cook until bubbling. Whisk in the milk slowly and bring to a gentle boil. Simmer for three minutes. Whisk in the cheese and stir until melted. Whisk in the mustard and sprinkle salt and pepper to taste. Whisk the egg yolks into this mixture and set aside. In a clean, dry bowl, beat the egg whites until stiff and add them in two batches to the soufflé mixture. Do not overmix, but fold the egg whites gently until well mixed. Pour into the glass dish and bake for twenty minutes. Serve immediately to the sound of loud applause. This is not a particularly puffy and elaborate souffle, but it tastes just like one. ⁂

wear more cashmere

AND FINALLY, AT LONG LAST, I WOULD VERY MUCH suggest that you wear more cashmere. Treat yourself often to the luxury fabric that has been described as "softness straight from heaven." Yes, it is self-indulgent, but after all of this, you know you deserve it. Because world production is so small, cashmere is a luxury fiber. China, Mongolia, Iran, Afghanistan, Turkey, and the Indian subcontinent are just a few of the places where it is made from the downy undercoat of the Kashmir goat. Why do we all love cashmere so much? I think it is because of the draping quality, the way it seems to melt like butter on your skin and keep you toasty warm. Cashmere really is the same as pashmina, which swept through fashion circles a few years back as the must-have shawl. Of course, your bare shoulders should be draped in cashmere—how could they not be?

Remember, though, that "cashmere" is a wonderful metaphor for whatever it is that we seem to deny ourselves. "Oh no," you say, as someone offers you a treat, "I really shouldn't...." Yes, you really should. You really should treat yourself to the occasional indulgence, you really should construct your own world that looks the way you want it to, in which the things you love can easily be found. Why pour yourself and your energies into others on an endless basis? Please, save some of you for *you*. And I'll see you at the cashmere counter! ⟨⊀⟩

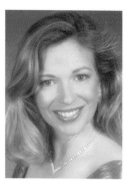

about the author

A longtime fan of small indulgences, cashmere-loving **Jennifer** (known to her friends as "Gin") **Sander** is the best-selling author of more than a dozen books, including the best-selling "Miracle Books" series for William Morrow. The busy mother of two boys, years ago she posted a small note on her computer to remind herself to "wear more cashmere," and the rest is history.

Jennifer and her books have been featured on "The View" with Barbara Walters, "American Journal," "C-Span's Book TV," "Fox and Friends," and "It's a Miracle." Articles about Jennifer have appeared in *USA Today*, *New York Newsday*, *Cosmopolitan* magazine, the *Boston Globe*, the *Los Angeles Times*, the *Sacramento Bee*, and many other magazines, newspapers, and television shows. A popular public speaker, she lives in northern California.

a note from the author

Well, are you ready to lead the cashmere life? Slip into your high-heel mules and join me as I further explore the many ways in which we can all feel special in our everyday lives. Sign up to receive my free *Wear More Cashmere* e-mail newsletter and I promise that, with this help, you will never be without an amusing friend to guide you through life's blander moments. Filled with more luxurious ideas about life, love, and lipstick (not to mention plenty of new ways you can feel like suburban royalty), you can sign up for the newsletter at www.wearmorecashmere.com. Visit today and learn about how you can throw a *Wear More Cashmere* party for your closest friends. Hmmm, sounds delicious... whatever will you wear?

Keep wearing cashmere,
Jennifer "Gin" Sander